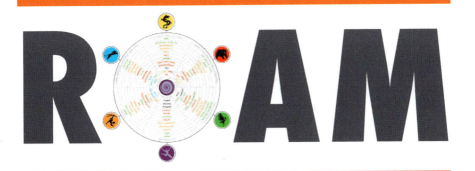

MOVEMENT AS MEDICINE

ROAM stands for Range of Active Movement and is an East meets West exercise guide that helps you improve your freedom of movement and your ability to move in a safe, progressive and enjoyable way.

ROAM: Movement as Medicine
by Ross Eathorne

Copyright © 2016 Ross Eathorne

All rights reserved. This book was self-published by Ross Eathorne. No part of this book may be reproduced in any form by any means without the express permission of the author. This includes reprints, excerpts, photocopying, recording, or any future means of reproducing text.

ISBN-13: 978-9881463838

ISBN-10: 9881463831

Printed by CreateSpace, An Amazon.com Company

CONTENTS

Dedication   v
Summary   vii
Also by the Author   ix
Preface   xi
Introduction   xv

ROAM   3

MOVEMENT AS MEDICINE   13
    1. Restoring Your Health   15
    2. Compliance, The Modern Dilemma of Movement   19
    3. ROAM: An Entertraining Coaching Method   23
    4. Goals, Benefits, and the Method   27
    5. Life Movements and Five-Animal Fitness   31
    6. Identifying Your Power Animal   35
    7. The Journey of Man   41
    8. Vitruvian Man and Fascial Lines   47
    9. Restoration Begins With Posture   53
    10. Squat Like a Tiger   61
    11. Twist Like a Dragon   69
    10. Bend Like a Bear   77
    11. Push Like a Crane   83
    12. Pull Like a Monkey   91

Author's note   99
Bibliography   103

"You can learn more about a person
in an hour of exercise
than in a year of
conversation"

Plato

DEDICATION

Mrs Hyndman (deceased) from Nae Nae intermediate (aged 11) who cornered me in the playground and insisted I enter the "A" grade gymnastics competition (when I had been avoiding gymnastics in favour of Hutt Valley representative rugby). To my surprise I went onto win the competition. I thank her for her vision.

All the gymnastics coaches I have been in contact with - parent helpers, Olympic and World Champion coaches. Greg Hammond, Kylie Carter, Arlene Thomas and Ruth Pirihi my sport aerobic coaches who took this rugby playing gymnast with no sense of music, rhythm, dance or stage presentation and patiently put together Sport Aerobic routines that enabled me to represent New Zealand at 10 World Championships and along the way win Two World Mr Fitness titles.

Grahame Eathorne (my dad) my first Rugby and Sailing coach for his knowledge of street sports psychology and the lessons of skill acquisition he gave.

To Bronwyn Cooper for whom I would have been lost to the fitness industry in 1996 if she had not brought back a Swiss ball from a conference and introduced me to functional fitness and Paul Chek.

To Glen Small who showed me that reading references and resources really brought deep understanding of a subject.

To Paul Chek who I learnt the patterns, rules and strategy of exercise kinesiology from.

To Frank Forencich who gave me courage to throw the rule book out the window in favour of play.

To Kit Laughlin Posture and flexibility guru who said to look for the original source.

And all my gymnasts, clients and mini rugby players that have helped me refine my craft and gave me the opportunity to develop and action my ideas.

SUMMARY

As modern day life becomes more convenient, movement has become less necessary. Ease and convenience are even seen as signs of success. At the same time, never has there been so much discussion about health and wellbeing as there is today, yet our desire for ease is driving us further from achieving an active life, proven to be associated with health.

Here is a book about re-engaging with our bodies to re-activate our full range of natural movement. It covers how both body and mind benefit by going back to our innate range of motions, where ideas about health have gone off-track, and how to get physical activity back into your life in a way that suits you. Ross Eathorne takes his experiences as a L.I.F.E (Lifestyle, Intention, Food, Exercise) Practitioner, drawing on a balance of Eastern and Western practices to show us how we can harness movement as medicine to improve our health, fitness and performance levels - physically, emotionally, mentally and spiritually.

Movement as Medicine is a guide. It takes us through self-assessments and step-by-step illustrated movement patterns. Eathorne explains the theory and techniques of his five animal fitness system that activates a variety of foundational body movements. You decide how and at what level to incorporate the movements into your lifestyle, but whether you are an athlete, a beginner or somewhere in between, there's something for anyone who has ever wondered about a lifelong health and fitness programme.

Dip into this insightful and practical book to restore your body to its natural state -- through fluid movement and mobility -- for lifelong health.

ALSO BY THE AUTHOR

Parts of *Movement as Medicine*, *The YogaVinQi Code* and *ROAM* have been adapted into iOS apps for the Apple iPhone:

Bodyweight Ninja is a dynamic warm-up routine, moving the body according to the way it was designed to move. Performed at a faster pace, it is an effective warm-up for sports and physical activity. It can be used as a bodyweight workout for active recovery days. Performed at a slower pace, it helps restore the body and calm the mind. It includes optional animal crawls and balance poses. This is my first iOS app, and it is available for free download on the App Store.

5-Animal Mobility provides a similar format to the animal exercise series, focusing on movement and mobility. This app includes high-quality Before, During, and After photos, detailed written instructions, and full video clips of the stretches and movements.

Bodyweight Ninja 90 is a 90-day progressive fitness programme including cardio, rest and lifestyle suggestions. This bodyweight programme has beginner, intermediate and advanced options. The first 30-day phase provides a foundation of mobility and movement patterns together with cardio development. The second and third 30-day phases increase the mobility, intensity, complexity and integration of the movement patterns to raise the metabolism in order to burn fat. There is plenty of variety offered, with more than 40 restoration and training sessions and more than 10 cardio sessions for the beginner and intermediate levels. The advanced level has 45 resistance sessions and 25 cardio sessions. The time of sessions varies greatly, from 5 minutes to 60 minutes post warm-up, depending on your fitness level and the effort and rest you require when completing the challenges.

Also by the Author

Calm Your Mind offers some short and long term strategies to calm your mind.

The Bottom Line of Fat Loss takes a holistic approach to fat loss, and turns over every grey stone to the bottom line of what is needed to loose fat and keep it off for life.

PREFACE

When an animal experiences stress, a survival reflex releases a dose of adrenaline into the bloodstream, eliciting one of three responses. Fight: never get caught between the river and the cub of a female hippopotamus! Flight: a wildebeest is very skittish and runs away at the drop of a hat. Freeze: a lizard relies on its camouflage to protect itself from danger.

Humans experience the same adrenaline release in response to stress. However, unlike an animal (for example, a dog will run away, find somewhere safe to hide, and discharge stress by panting), humans can choose to ignore the stress. Ignoring stress does not discharge the chemical reaction, and these chemicals are stored in our bodies according to the nature of the stress.

If the stress is physical trauma, then the stress is centred on the impact site. If it is hormonal stress (from an unbalanced diet, for instance) then the gland which issues the hormone becomes stressed from overwork. If it is emotional stress induced by anxiety, this will affect the organ related to anxiety, according to Traditional Chinese Medicine (which I will refer to hereafter as TCM). If it is mental stress accumulated from having too much on your plate, your brain will refuse to shut down at night, resulting in insomnia. Lack of sleep affects all other systems, resulting in a complicated mess of low energy, pain, and illness. An excess of stress stored in the body may cause you to develop autoimmune disease.

Movement as Medicine restores calmness to the body, mind and spirit through the power of intention, specific exercises, and breathwork.

The intention comes from TCM's five-element theory and each element's corresponding positive emotions. The specific exercises are full yoga asanas that move the body according to its three-dimensional architecture and are mapped according to Chinese meridian and Western fascial lines. The breath connects the body and mind and manifests in spirit.

Meditation, Qigong, tai chi and yoga are good outlets for releasing stress because they are performed in serene places, accompanied by calm music, and are based around breathing. The focus is on the here and now, not on what has happened or will happen. Posing and moving increases the circulation, releases tension, and improves the stability of muscles and joints.

Yoga asanas help to stretch and stabilise joints and muscles via the intake and outflow of breath. Each of these poses either stimulates or sedates a specific chakra and its affiliated organ, hormone, and emotion. Yoga is the union of the body, mind and spirit, as are qigong, tai chi, and any movement done at an easy pace, in time with the breath. Yogis put themselves in certain positions in order to understand the workings of the world around them. By doing so, they gain empathy, compassion and sensitivity, qualities that elevate the state of mind.

I have distilled my understanding of yoga; Western anatomy, movement systems, and medical healing; and qigong into 5 yoga asanas, 5 yoga balancing poses, and the intention to hold in your mind's eye as you count your breaths. The intention is the positive emotion of TCM's Five-Element Theory.

Medicine: Something that affects well-being
Well-being: The state of being happy, healthy or prosperous.
(Merriam-Webster.com)

Movement as Medicine develops your well-being by using exercise and intention to balance the body and mind.

As I have gotten older, I have realised that there is no "best" way to solve a problem, achieve a task or break a record. Sadly, many within the fitness industry are adamant that their way (or their charismatic guru's way) is the only way, and that others are inferior and wrong. I myself have, in the past, perpetuated this folly of youth; however, these days, I feel concerned about the person who seeks to force his opinion before first seeking to understand and then to figure out how to employ this understanding.

In 2010, during a taxi ride in Bangalore, India, I discussed this industry problem with my driver, who turned out to be a Doctor of Philosophy. He replied with this wisdom: "We all do the same thing; we all belong to the same circle; the problem is that we do the same thing differently and come at it from different angles."

Since then, I have compared Western exercise science, movement systems, and psychology with Eastern wisdom and movement systems. *Movement as Medicine* and *The YogaVinQi Code* compare the two, drawing parallels wherever possible, and strive to use the best of both worlds to improve your health, in order to enable your happiness and prosperity.

This book is about preventing chronic injury caused by overuse of certain movement patterns that lead to muscle imbalance and poor posture; and restoring the body after such an injury. Acute trauma-induced injury requires intensive, one-on-one professional care.

Enjoying regular and varied exercise is the key to achieving lifelong health, fitness and performance. Enjoyment motivates you to repeat the experience. Regularity ensures fitness and skill development. Variety prevents you from becoming bored. It is important to provide a constant supply of new stimulus to which the body will adapt, in turn promoting further enjoyment, fitness, and skill development. The aim is to perpetuate the habit of this enjoyment-adaptation cycle.

Exercise once a week and you will go backwards; twice a week, and you will stay the same; more than three times a week, and you will progress. This adage is applicable to any skill development. Exercising three times a week for a month will result in significant change—you will receive compliments from people who have not seen you for a while. If you exercise three times a week for three months, you'll observe a significant change in how you look and feel. Regular training for three months may empower you to focus on a skill set and to participate in a physical adventure or sport competition, such as a challenging hike or an obstacle race.

Generally speaking, people restarting fitness training will take around six weeks to adapt to any specified exercise. People with around two years of regular fitness training will take around four weeks to adapt. Athletes with many years of experience will take two weeks to adapt.

Adaptation is the enemy of progress. Once the body has adapted, it is no longer being stimulated. The body has become efficient, so there will be neither a decrease in fat nor an increase in muscle tone or skill. If you continue to do what you have always done, the muscles responsible for performing a specific task will become overused at around the three-month mark (if not sooner) and this leads to injury. Varying the volume, intensity, time and type of training within your three-plus sessions per week and in your experience bracket (2, 4 or 6 weeks) will ensure continued stimulus and growth as well as helping you to avoid burnout and injury.

Therefore, variety is the key to continued stimulation of psychological and physiological enjoyment, and encourages the sedentary majority to improve its health and fitness. There are infinite ways to stimulate the body and mind to promote growth; the trick is to make it large enough to get satisfactory gains and small enough not to overdo it.

Many people aim for large gains, biting off more than they can chew. They may follow a programme they've seen on the Internet or in a magazine that shows only an end phase—the "sexy" programme—and not the weeks, months or years of preparation preceding it. Doing so may lead to injury.

INTRODUCTION

I grew up in New Zealand. For most of my childhood, my backyard was native bush—an adventure playground where my friends and I could enjoy creek jumping, tree and waterfall climbing, sheep chasing, and exploring, free of the threat that any animal could attack, bite or poison us. In winter, we played rugby and soccer on the neighbour's lawn; in summer, cricket in our quiet cul-de-sac. My climbing skills and sense of adventure led me to gain national representative honours in gymnastics, and, once earned, those skills returned me to the rugby field for senior and provincial-level honours. Along the way, I sailed in the windy waters of Wellington; swam, biked and ran many triathlons; and dragon-boated for a corporate team.

My movement scenario (with a few tweaks) is commonplace in New Zealand, where there is an abundance of opportunity available to everyone. After living in Hong Kong for thirteen years and raising three children here, I can say that, by far, this city offers far fewer movement opportunities. Many of the spontaneous activities have been replaced by structured activities. Initially, my kids would exercise only through scheduled, paid-for activities, complete with a uniform and a medal awarded after each class. I have observed that many Hong Kong children are overscheduled. There is little opportunity for unscheduled, unstructured play. This breaks my heart.

Equally, adults may overschedule one type of movement pattern (golf or running, for example) to the extent that it leads to injury and burnout. In my own approach to training for an event, I have at times become so focused on the mechanics and physiological science of programme design that I ended up squeezing all the joy out of the activity. The over-achievement focus is so intense that the spirit of why we do sport (for challenge, enjoyment, camaraderie, health, and fitness) becomes lost. Overdosing on movement can transform it from a medicine into a poison.

Movement as Medicine is the first level of helping to restore health (the absence of disease) through movement and intention. This book covers the inner, mostly

INTRODUCTION **XV**

red-coloured concentric circles up to the Crawl-Coordination level of the Range of Motion circle.

I travel around Asia lecturing on health, fitness and performance, and I draw on the principles of Qigong in my movement lectures. Qigong is the integration of physical posture, breathing technique, and focused intention. *Qi* means life force, and *gong* means skill cultivated through steady practice. I divide the groups into five movement types—*squat, twist, bend, push,* and *pull*—and assign an animal to each movement. I explain that various tai chi schools in China assign each of the five elements—Wood, Fire, Earth, Metal and Water—with an animal that best represents its characteristics.

There is no universal matching of animals to elements, and they vary from one school to another. An animal may represent Water in one school and Earth in another. If you think about the Famous Five in the movie *Kung Fu Panda*, you are on the right track, except that TCM and its branch of medical Qigong is very complex. It requires decades of study to gain a full understanding of it and to reach the title of master.

Those in the East want to know more about the West, and those in the West want to know more about the East. While I have taken my formal and industry education from the West, I have been based in Hong Kong since 2003, and have developed my lectures and, subsequently, this book as a bridge between the East and the West.

There are a billion Chinese people on the planet. Of these, 7 million (predominantly Cantonese) live in Hong Kong. Many Chinese people practice feng shui, a system of placing yourself in harmony with your environment. To this end, the majority of Hong Kong's buildings face north, and many apartment buildings situated near mountains (which signify dragons) contain empty spaces within their structure, in order to allow the dragons access to and from their lairs.

A few years ago, when I first became curious about qi, I brought some friends to Middle Island Yacht Club for dinner and pointed out such a gap in a building in the adjacent Repulse Bay. When I asked them what they thought about it, one of them, an architect from Hungary, dismissed its mystical purpose, saying that it had a practical function—to decrease the effect of strong winds during typhoon season. I was a little put out by her response, as, after living for two years in Hong Kong, I knew people who had shifted apartments and offices according to feng shui. Mothers elect to give birth by C-section on auspicious dates; and people check the birthdates of their prospective business partners to see if the match will bring good luck. Now, I realise there is not need to be put off as it is just another example of someone looking at the same thing differently.

The chinese put a gap in a structure to allow the dragon access, whereas the western architects rationalise putting a gap in a building in a place known for its typhoons is a practical and sensible thing to do. Same thing but different.

Chinese numerology demonstrates the power behind the belief system of qi. The number 8 is similar to the infinity symbol; the Chinese word for eight sounds similar to the word for prosper; and there is a resemblance between the Chinese characters for 88 and for double happiness. Reflect upon this for a moment: Is this due to coincidence, public relations, or strong belief that the opening ceremony of the Summer Olympics in Beijing began on the eighth day of the eighth month of the year 2008, at eight minutes and eight seconds past eight o'clock in the evening?

Which processes did the Chinese carry out, over how long a period of time, and with which populations and controls, to uncover these strong beliefs? It's a mindboggling question, and perhaps a scientist or an architect could outline its feasibility. All I know is that there must be something to this force called qi. I have aimed to simplify my personal understanding of TCM, five-element theory, and Qigong exercises.

This brings me to yoga, the physical exercise and healing system developed in India at around the same time as, or perhaps slightly earlier than, Qigong. While there are some clear similarities between them—the Mountain Pose in yoga is virtually identical to the "Immortal Post" posture in qigong—I will be so bold as to say that yoga is biased to static holds, and pauses between a series of poses, whilst Qigong is biased toward cyclic movement that repeats itself for a prescribed time before transitioning to another movement. The primary similarity between them is that their movements are tuned to the breath.

I challenge you to perform once the Qi cultivation exercise of standing still with your arms extended in front of you, as though resting on a big bubble. My Qigong studies require this practice for between fifteen minutes and an hour each day. To those of my clients who have "monkey mind", I have recommended doing this for an hour a day, as one of the most difficult and yet beneficial holiday activities.

In yoga, a gymnastics scale balance or dancer's arabesque is called Warrior III. Upon realising this, I looked back at all the movement systems I had learned over the years: gymnastics, Kit Laughlin's Posture & Flexibility, Paul Chek's Primal Movement Patterns, Thomas Myers' Anatomy Trains, TRX Suspension Training, ViPR Loaded Movement Training, Trigger Point Performance Therapy and SMRT-CORE, DNS (Dynamic Neuromuscular Stability), and Pavigym, to name a few. Yoga postures can be seen in all of these systems, which are arguably derived from yoga. Further investigation showed various yoga postures corrected muscle imbalances, unblocked illnesses, and engaged or enhanced bodily functions. Yoga poses can be broken down from full (high level of difficulty) asanas to their subsets (individual muscles of each fascial line). Yoga is more than a physical system of healing; it has emotional and spiritual healing properties.

Well-being is the state of being happy, healthy or prosperous, and achieving this state is the aim of *Movement as Medicine*. At the very least, doing one or all of the stretches will release body tension; at best, steady practise of the stretches, posture exercises, and appropriate intentions will allow the well-being of body, mind and spirit.

Movement as Medicine is about balancing the body and mind with exercise and intention. The primary aim is to restore posture and fluidity of movement. All exercises are of low-to- moderate intensity. You may opt to skip an exercise, as doing some exercise is better than doing none at all.

To gong or not to gong?

Small improvements in your well-being can be gained by performing one of the exercises for as few as five breaths per day. Significant changes in well-being can be attained by carrying out only one step, or all five, in the cycle of what the Chinese call a *gong*. A gong (or practice) can last a hundred consecutive days. It's up to you how long you invest.

Movement as Medicine's secondary aim is to prepare you for the progression from health to fitness. Fitness training, strength and work capacity of moderate to high intensity exercise is hacked in my book ROAM (which stands for Range of Active Movement).

So, why aren't we happy, healthy and prosperous?

I have met many people we might call prosperous, many of whom are not truly happy, and many of whom are far from healthy. In many cases, the cause lies in the very pursuit of prosperity. You spend so much time chasing money and brokering business deals that your outlook narrows and your priorities blur. Before you know it, fifteen years have passed and your kids have grown up. Your girth has expanded, your back aches, you often feel bloated, tired, grumpy, and irrational. You know that exercise will help to improve your well-being, but you are pressed for time and have grown bored of the tricep pushdown, the treadmill, and the gym. You are not alone in this dilemma.

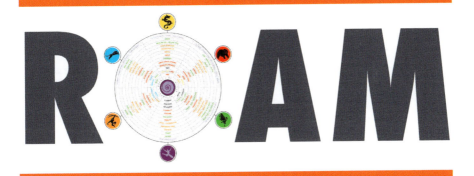

MOVEMENT AS MEDICINE

ROAM stands for Range of Active Movement and is an East meets West exercise guide that helps you improve your freedom of movement and your ability to move in a safe, progressive and enjoyable way.

ROAM

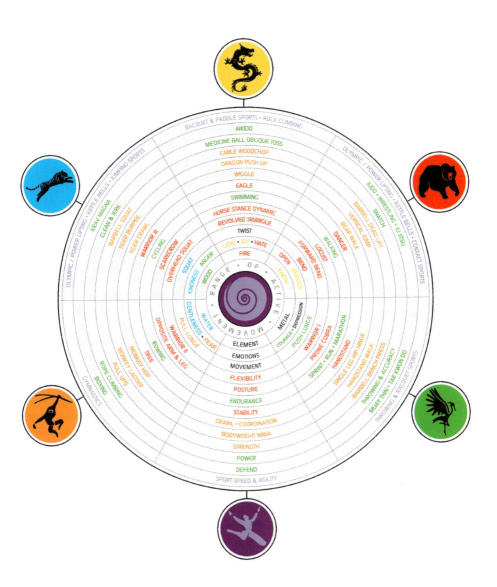

ROAM: MOVEMENT AS MEDICINE

4   ROAM: MOVEMENT AS MEDICINE

What is ROAM?

Range

Of

Active

Movement.

The aim of ROAM is to increase your ability to move. You can roam across a broad landscape of movement patterns and modalities - bodyweight, stability ball, suspension training, elastic bands, cables, dumbbells, barbells, kettle bells, medicine balls, sandbags and so on - in a random manner to increase your general fitness and stay in shape. This is called general physical preparation (GPP) as represented by the spiral development pattern in ROAM cycle centre. Or you can train specific physical preparation (SPP) by focusing on sport performance movement patterns and abilities as represented by one of the animal wedges in the cycle.

In May of 2015 I started to train professional boxer, Rex Tso. I didn't know anything about the specifics of boxing at the time but I did know about energy systems, movement analysis and programme design. My summation of Rex was that he was fit and fast inside the ring but he was not very flexible nor did he move well outside of the ring. 12 months later Rex returned from a month long training camp and started our normal dynamic warm-up; I commented that it was noticeable he was moving with much more fluidity now. He smiled and said that he had taken a young professional boxer through our warm-up and specific stretching routine and he had seen how stiff, awkward and uncomfortable the rookie was during the session, just like he had been 12 months ago. The rookie provided a mirror image of how far he had progressed. At this point I told Rex he had been transformed in a year from a boxer to an athlete and as a result was now a better boxer. Rex's training is high-end, meaning six days a week, three sessions per day of conditioning, cardio and boxing training and you can even count massage, sleeping during the day and stretching at night. When he has a "fight in sight" we concentrate on specific physical conditioning for boxing and when he has an off-season we do general physical conditioning to add a broader movement ability to his arsenal.

ROAM has the ability to cycle around broad movements and also to focus in on specific movements. The beauty of ROAM is that it is designed to stimulate everyone - from professional athletes to children - to enjoy, regular and varied exercise.

Life movement

Most movements in life and sport can be distilled into six movements patterns plus gait (walking, running). I call these "Life Movements". Others call them primal, foundation, fundamental movement patterns and they are represented by the squat, twist, bend, push, pull and lunge.

The basic premise of ROAM is to spiral around the life movement patterns to develop ever increasing competencies of flexibility, stability, endurance, strength, coordination, power, speed, agility, infant developmental crawling, throwing, accuracy, defence and sport performance. The end goal is the ability to roam free, to enable all the competencies available to man (represented by the Leaping Man icon) and to be able to execute them according to the opportunities and obstacles presented by a sporting or natural environment. This end goal I attribute to George Hebert, founder of Method Natural "Be strong to be useful" which provides an altruistic purpose for a fitness practise.

East meets West

Traditional Chinese Medicine's (TCM) five element theory and Yoga movement practices have physical-mental-emotional and spiritual qualities that are beyond the scope of this book. I have assimilated them using one of five elements, a positive and negative emotion and an animal that expresses these qualities in its movements and personality. Likewise, humans often express their mindset by the movement choices or sports they do; spend a week at the Olympic Games and you can see a trend of personality, body shape, posture and movement abilities for specific sports. In ROAM East represents wisdom, emotion, creativity and stuff that can't be measured. West represents science, logic, structure and everything that can be measured.

X factor

George Hebert states exercise above all metrics needs to be enjoyable and I agree with him. An Olympic champion or athlete who stands atop of the dias in any sport is often said to have the "X factor" which is a non-quantifiable separation from second and third place getters. What is the difference, when most people in the top 10 train in almost exactly the same way? I offer this explanation: the person performs without thinking and beyond any textbook. They operates in the zone of optimal performance with a calm mind and in a state of Zen or enlightenment.

Concentric circles of Health, Fitness and Performance

ROAM, or range of active movement, expands in concentric circles. Each layer expands your movement periphery and ability to move. Put another way, each circle increases your ability to perform and play with anyone at any time. ROAM has three phases:

1.Health

Moshen Feldenkrais said "All movement begins and ends in posture". Posture is the realm of health. Health is defined as the absence of disease. The first seven rings are aimed at restoring posture and basic movement mechanics using low intensity, bodyweight stretches and activation exercises. Several rings are coloured red as it is critical they are performed correctly in order to reduce the risk of injury before you progress to the crawl, bodyweight ninja and strength intensity rings. Each animal strength exercise has a cardiovascular endurance modality assigned - e.g. green is the colour of the lungs. Movement as Medicine is focused on these levels.

2. Fitness

The amber rings represent a jump up in complexity and intensity of movements. Exercises in the fitness phase boost metabolism and are designed to develop strength and coordination. The fitness phase is where the strength meets function. This is where we add equipment to bodyweight movement competencies. The equipment or modalities I favour are stability balls, suspension trainers, elastic resistance, cables, dumbbells, barbells, kettle bells, medicine balls, ropes, sandbags and sleds. One who is grounded in bodyweight basics need not limit themselves to any one modality and should be adaptable enough to create exercise with whatever is at hand and whatever they think is the best tool for a specific purpose. The strength exercise for the Tiger, Bear and Crane focuses on the strength and conditioning "gold standard" lifts of squat, deadlift and bench press (these three lifts are competed for in the sport of powerlifting). The cable reverse woodchopper and the pull-up are the strength expressions of the Dragon and Monkey respectively. The strength levels are an exponential step up from bodyweight exercises and represent many accessory exercises to correct any weakness, isolate and integrate any muscles and overlap with the restoration phase.

Each circle lays a foundation step for the next circle.

3. Performance

The green rings are an accumulation of fitness abilities. This give the green light to put them into high intensity real-world scenarios of a defence style or sports performance. At the performance level there will be one dominant movement pattern but in reality many of the movement patterns will be used. For example the Monkey has great agility and as he swings through the trees he uses movements needed in boxing and gymnastic sports. Boxing, like gymnastics, requires greater agility but a punch also requires a powerful twist and push that comes from a strong lunge. so boxers must borrow exercises from the Dragon and Crane. The "X factor" throws the rule book out the window and creates it own rules.

Everyone performs, not everyone competes or likes to compete

First and foremost ROAM was developed for people who do not like to compete or participate in sports. It was developed to entertain people while they tone up and lose weight and at the same time give a purpose or theme to each session. It provides a cornucopia of movement variety and develops freedom and the ability to move.

To stay in shape and lose weight the body needs to be continually challenged and progressively overloaded. This means you need to puff a little, burn your muscles a little and every now and again have muscle soreness the next day. Why not satisfy these things while doing random workouts not focused on a sport?

A basic ROAM cycle is:

First day	squat themed session
Second day	twist themed session
Third day	bend themed session
Fourth & Fifth Days	Crane and Monkey session

You can rest during the weekend or perform a session where you mix up all themes in an obstacle course such as Parkour, Spartan or Tough Mudder.

Leaping Man is the key

The legend of ROAM's movement abilities can be found above the Leaping Man icon. Each title is a theme of that circle and is represented in an archetype of each animal. Understanding the themes unlocks multiple ways the ROAM cycle can be used. A skilled practitioner can tailor an exercise programme to suit their particular ambition, conditions, ability and circumstance. I caution a totally random approach until you have developed at least one full spiral of movement competencies to a performance level. In my experience a shortcut

8 ROAM: MOVEMENT AS MEDICINE

in exercise usually results in a technique that breaks down under pressure and results in injury. Inevitably restoration can take the same amount of time, or longer, to achieve than if they had not taken the short-cut in the first place. For the inexperienced, the best place to start is with structure. With Rex we were able to fill in his movement gaps because we played with the life movement patterns and expanded his range of active movement. Rex's increased ability to move broadened his base of conditioning and allowed him to reach higher sport-specific peaks when fight night came along.

When you drop a pebble in a still pond the waves expand in concentric circles: they do not flow in predication triangles, nor do they have multiple starting points. The starting point is the centre. It is likely that you will be really good at one of the Life Movement patterns, bad at another and a mixture good and bad at the rest. As humans we tend to stick to what we do best and what make us feel better and neglect what we can't do, yet is critical for us to prevent injury and do exercise that completes us as movers. When we start at the centre and spiral out, visiting each movement pattern as per the concentric circle theme, we discover the gaps in our movement abilities and have the opportunity to work on our weaknesses with accessory exercises.

Flexibility

The starting point of ROAM's movement is a yoga asana. The yoga asana expresses that life movement's full range of active movement. The yoga pose also represents a scaling of that asana into 8-13 separate isolated muscles stretches that we added together to create a synergy, fluidity and great ROAM. The pose includes a dominant fascial line, a meridian line, one of the five elements, a positive and negative emotion - a chakra with a physical-mental-emotional-spiritual metaphysical lesson (outlined in more detail in "The YogaVinQi Code").

Endurance

Cardiovascular efficiency is one of the biggest foundations for fitness as it helps to circulate nutrients and oxygen around the body and to remove waste products. The cardio modality assigned is flexible and can easily be swapped with other animals. Postural endurance is another goal in the health phase.

Stability

Flexibility without stability leads to speed wobbles and injury. Most people are weak in the frontal or side-to-side plane of movement. To counter this, each animal has a single leg stability pose. The exception is the Crane which has the handstand - an advanced pose. Stability also means activation of movement-specific muscles in a whole-part-whole format. Flexibility with stability is called mobility and is the major benefit of ROAM, Movement as Medicine, as it provides flexibility, stability and an activation exercise series for each life movement.

Crawl - Coordination.

There are a lot more crawl patterns than the five presented in ROAM. Ask any recreational gymnastic coach and they could teach you a zoo full. These crawl patterns originated from infant developmental patterns and require full integration of life movement-specific brain power and muscles. I use the crawl patterns to assimilate the extra range of motion of the stretches and activation exercises.

Bodyweight Ninja

The aim of Bodyweight Ninja is to construct a body that can operate at a high level of movement and prepare it for the dangers of external load. The culmination of the bodyweight inner rings is a high-intensity expression of the animal using bodyweight only.

Strength

The barbell exercises best represent strength training goals. The circle of strength is where we introduce equipment to both regress with accessory exercise and progress towards power and Olympic lifting exercises.

Power, Throwing & Accuracy

Power is moving things quickly, gathering and using momentum. Power is a performance realm. An unconditioned, immobile body cannot control the forces and this takes the joints past their flexibility range and causes impingement and soft tissue trauma. Throwing a great distance requires power. Accuracy is a skill and requires practice to acquire.

Defend

There are many self-defence/fighting disciplines to choose from and you could argue which animal qualities fit what style. I present my rationale for each style and animal qualities below. I am an expert at none of them.

1. Tiger - Krav Maga: A Tiger is quick and powerful and an encounter with one is over quickly. Krav Maga is an Israeli self defence style that aims to stop a fight as soon as possible.

2. Dragon - Aikido: A Dragon is a magical, mystical creature that twists and turns. Aikido uses clever twists and turns and body locks to immobilise opponents.

3. Bear- Judo - Wrestling- Ju jitsu: A bear is big and strong, is able to stand on two feet but is strongest on the ground. Judo, wrestling and ju jitsu start on the ground but the winning of a fight comes on the ground.

4. Crane - Muay Thai - Tae Kwon Do: A Crane has long legs that enables it to walk in swamps, Cranes often wait for their prey perched on one leg. Muay Thai and Tae Kwon Do are kickboxing sports that require great leg flexibility.

Sport Speed & Agility

Different sports require different forms of speed: boxers require hand speed, sprinters leg speed and so on. Agility is the ability to change direction and is one of the most difficult skills to acquire. It needs joint stability, strength, power, speed and the ability to remain injury-free from when executing a move. These sports are the full expression of a life movement pattern. At this level of performance other movement patterns should be introduced as they will contribute more and more.

Play

"When you play you fill in the gaps that structure doesn't find".

Overall, the essence of ROAM is to play. The leaping man combines all the movement patterns, abilities and physiology into one symbol of play. ROAM does provide a structure to help you revive, restore and recreate your ability to play, at whatever level of engagement you want until you can throw the rule book away and create your own ones. I do suggest for safety and competency that complete one cycle of the animal series in this book, perhaps following along in the iPhone app to find your gaps and develop them, then progress onto different mobilities and the ever increasing complexity and intensities of the outer rings to keep your play close to your conditioning and ability levels.

At certain level of play can be had by imagining being your power, critical or any animal for that matter when doing your movement habit. You could do the particular animal series with the positive emotion as your intention and see how that lifts your mood.

ROAM - Movement as Medicine is at the bodyweight level. It offers five series of flexibility, stability and life movement activation exercises to help you revive, restore and recreate your exercise habit. There is not much "play" in this book: it is more about paving the way for the fitness level where you take function and add strength, coordination and equipment.

Inside you will find out how to identify your:

1. Power animal: the yoga asana and life movement pattern that you are most fluid with, grounds you and empowers you to feel good about yourself.

2. Critical animal: it is critical to develop the most restricted asana because exercises in that life movement pattern, especially with external load and speed, are likely to lead to an injury.

Why ROAM, Movement as Medicine, is also a book for:

Beginners:

- Exercises employ your own body weight, removing the obstacle of purchasing equipment and gym membership
- Exercise complexity and intensity are calibrated for deconditioned or returning-to-fitness levels
- Assessments are simple and progress becomes self-evident
- Increases your life movement ability and provides a foundation for further functional and strength fitness training
- Each movement has specific health benefits particularly when used in conjunction with the positive emotion.

Those who become easily bored:

- The variety keeps your body challenged and your mind fresh.
- Those with limited time:
- All the exercise thinking has been done for you.
- One is better than none. You can choose to do as many exercises as you have time for.

This is a movement book primarily focused on improving your ability to perform functional movement from scratch. It presents five series of stretch, mobility and balance exercises and gives a simple assessment so you can identify the movement that you most need to do in order to balance your posture, reduce risk of injury, and increase your ability to move.

12   ROAM: MOVEMENT AS MEDICINE

MOVEMENT AS MEDICINE

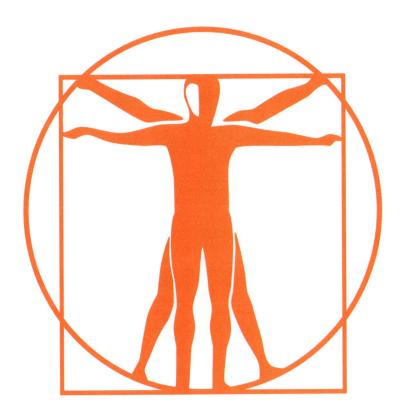

14   ROAM: MOVEMENT AS MEDICINE

1. Restoring Your Health

"Health is the new wealth." –Unattributed

Health is the absence of disease

We can combine the static and dynamic yoga and Qigong postures with the three-dimensional science, anatomy and architecture of the Vitruvian Man, with the aim of cultivating life force and healing, restoring freedom of motion, and providing a safe (whole-part-whole) method of progressing a person's exercise experience.

The YogaVinQi Code is the rationale behind my *Bodyweight Ninja, 5-Animal Mobility* and *Bodyweight Ninja 90* fitness apps for iPhone, which offer the following benefits:

- Restores freedom of motion in a specific joint, muscle or movement, and indeed to the whole body

- Encourages the intention to replace a negative emotion with a positive one

- Stimulates the circulation of nutrients to and from organs, endocrine glands, and muscles

- Prevents injury by providing you with an appropriate warm-up, with emphasis on mobility and safe teaching progressions through low, moderate and high complexity and intensity exercise

- Provide a variety of bodyweight movement modalities to keep the exercise programme fresh, challenging and enjoyable

- Remove the barrier of having to purchase a gym membership

- After the bodyweight programmes, I plan to offer a programme based upon Five-Animal Mobility and utilising TRX suspension training, kettlebells, medicine balls, cables, dumbbells and free weights

The Vitruvian Man table (at the end of Part I) and the YogaVinQi Code table (near the end of Part II) provide a Western and Eastern overview of how all the LIFE (Lifestyle, Intention, Food, and Exercise) relationships are related in this book. The posture exercises are designed to safely get you started. The asanas are full and advanced yoga poses that double as quick assessments—if you think any of the five poses are beyond your current physical ability, then you have identified a weakness. You once had the flexibility to easily execute these poses, but your circumstances and environment have led to its loss. These restrictions point to places of potential injury.

Every movement is an assessment and every assessment is a movement

The whole-part-whole method allows every movement to be an assessment and every assessment to be a movement, allowing a person to gain awareness of what is restricted and needs restoring, and what is functional and can be enhanced with fitness and performance training.

TCM systems of Qigong and tai chi, and the Ayurvedic system of yoga are between three thousand and five thousand years old. These methods use movement to stimulate the sympathetic and parasympathetic nervous systems.

Playing it safe

When reconditioning your body, it pays to play safe by progressing in three phases of gradually increasing intensity, volume and complexity. I label these three phases of exercise progression *health, fitness,* and *performance.*

This chapter is concerned with health—essentially, "heal thyself"—and the low-intensity exercise that can help you to build energy reserves (as opposed to draining them) and which is ideally suited to accompany other important health modalities of detoxification of the liver, colon, stomach, and brain.

The health phase lays the foundation to build a solid platform for high metabolism exercises in the fitness and performance phases. There are many exercises to choose from and an infinite number of ways to present them.

I have chosen them from my Western exercise science education: Thomas Myers' Anatomy Trains, Paul Chek's Primal Movement Patterns, TCM meridian lines, Qigong exercises, yoga asanas, and condensed these into what I think is the fewest number of exercises to have the best overall long-term effect. The yoga poses are full asanas and you may need to consult an instructor to help break them down into more manageable partial asanas. I have developed an exercise app called Five-Animal Mobility that does all of this for you.

Restoration of posture and pain-free movement is the basic level of health

Once you become aware of your posture and gain freedom of motion through isolated stretching and strengthening exercises, you can safely increase the metabolic demand of exercise by adding movement complexity and intensity.

The fitness level is moderate intensity (around 60-80% of your maximum heart rate) exercise.

Movement as Medicine and *The YogaVinQi Code* are systems of dynamic and static exercise that uses the Western architectural approach to the musculoskeletal system and integrates this with the Eastern understanding of how movement affects the nervous system, internal organs, glands, and emotions for the purpose of restoring all of the following:

- posture

- freedom of motion

- fight and flight states to rest and digest states

- positive moods

- health

Both these systems combined represent the first eight rings of ROAM. The goal of ROAM is to provide a system of safe, progressive movements that increases your Range of Active Movement, whilst enabling you to enjoy regular and varied exercise. The remaining rings of ROAM take a significant jump upwards in intensity and complexity, and these will be presented in my next book, *ROAM II: Function meets Strength.*

18   ROAM: MOVEMENT AS MEDICINE

2. Compliance, The Modern Dilemma of Movement

Gyms can be intimidating and overwhelming places, and programmes can be boring. All of this can be made worse when a person is out of condition, hasn't exercised for a while, and is apprehensive because of a previous injury. All of these factors may reduce exercise adherence (which impacts results) or prevent a person from starting to exercise in the first place.

Since 1993, I have worked as a personal trainer, coach, facilitator, guide and mentor in lifestyle, intention, food, exercise and movement; and before that, I competed in gymnastics, rugby, sailing, cricket, and other sports. I've identified the main reason for lack of results as being compliance, or consistency of practice. Fluidity comes from muscle memory; elasticity of muscles from regular mobilising and stretching; coordination, muscle tone, and injury correction all come from practice.

Time and inclination are the biggest obstacles I have to factor in when I negotiate, trick, scare, bully, cajole, persuade and motivate my clients to comply with any lifestyle, intention, food and exercise plan I design for them. This does not apply to all of my clients all of the time, but sometimes it sure feels like it. I coach housewives, CEOs, bankers, partners, students, and full-time athletes, all of whom have different life circumstances pulling them in different directions and which may override or govern their priorities. They all have different ambitions ranging from doing the bare minimum in order to keep a modicum of health and fitness to winning world titles, and varying conditions of posture, injury, and function; and they each bring with them broad physical abilities of past experiences—each client is unique in this regard.

All of us have the same amount of time. The way in which we schedule our time varies according to our priorities, values, and purpose, and this is called our lifestyle. Inclination to exercise gets sucked out of people because of how modern life makes demands on their time. Other factors include cost-benefit, return on investment, the intimidation of going to the gym alone, and feeling overwhelmed by the sheer volume of information, equipment, techniques and philosophies available in the health and fitness industry.

A big part of my role as a coach is to find ways around the obstacles listed above. The longer I can keep my clients motivated to exercise, the more likely they are to improve their well-being. When gyms do not regularly change their programmes, some of their patrons become bored. Some people give up and go to the pub instead, while others jump from one fitness trend to another. Another problem arises when people attempt to make too big a jump or too fast a progression in an effort to get to the sexy-level exercise and intensity. This is when injuries and burnout occur. Such shortcuts turn into a long way around, and rehabilitation proves more tedious than following a safer and more appropriate path.

So how can you or your trainer identify the appropriate level of exercise for you?

Answer this question: *What do you want?*

Spanish-based fitness company Pavigym recently published these statistics:

Why people exercise:

1.	To improve health	62%
2.	To improve fitness	40%
3.	To relax	36%
4.	To have fun	30%
5.	To control weight	24%
6.	To improve physical performance	24%

I divided these statistics into three progressive levels:

1. Health: You need to restore health because your condition is significantly impaired through of an injury or chronic disease.

2. Fitness: You want to improve your ability to build physical strength, functions and capacity.

3. Performance: You have the ambition and life circumstances to apply fitness at sport- specific intensity either in the gym or at an event.

Most people want to exercise just to improve health and fitness, to relax and have fun. Only 24% of people exercise to improve physical performance or control weight.

Sometimes life gets in the way of compliance. Your priorities change, and exercise, intention and nutrition sometimes have to take a back seat. I get that, but at what cost?

What if there was a simple system that took into account your life and minimised the cost, whilst allowing you the freedom to choose how much time to spend on it (from 5 breaths to 60 minutes); and offering a wide variety of exercises and equipment options (ranging from your own bodyweight, the portable and versatile TRX, kettlebells, and other gym-based equipment)? What if that system drew upon current Western science of movement mechanics and corrective exercise and the mind and spirit benefits of yoga and Qigong, and offered a safe, gradual progression of complexity and intensity to satisfy all reasons for exercising (and remove the obstacles to exercise)?

Movement as Medicine, and the ROAM cycle is that system.

I'd like to share a few case studies of clients who have helped me to develop this system over the last twenty-three years.

Susan
Susan had a couple of injuries but did not want to train in the main gym, because she was intimidated by its atmosphere, equipment and fit, Lycra-clad clientele. Instead, we went to a quiet area away from the main gym and used the TRX Suspension Trainer.

Alistair
Alistair is a company CEO I trained every two weeks, updating his programme and coaching him through it. Alistair was diligent with his self-practice, so I could progress him through a technically sound, linear path each training session. After a year or so, he had reached one of the highest levels of intensity and complexity in programming at the gym. Alistair told me that he liked three things in particular about our training.

1. I am a CEO and am responsible for driving the productivity and feedback of three hundred employees. You are the only person who gives me feedback.
2. Once every two weeks, for an hour, I don't have to think, as you do it all for me.
3. My PA and a few staff members know that I have been training with you, because my own productivity rises and I come back full of ideas and ready to delegate new business.

Neville

Neville, who holds an executive position at a bank, presented to me with a debilitating back injury. Over the course of a year, we significantly improved his quality of life and recreational activity. When we had built his pain-free function level to encompass almost all exercises, reaching what I would call the alpha level of intensity, Neville would score our workouts out of 10. If the score was below a 7, it was to me like a red rag to a bull, and Neville knew this. I would redouble my programme design to make sure that after the next session he would virtually crawl, exhausted, out of the gym. Although a very busy person, Neville made exercise a priority by having a regular appointment in the diary. He would even excuse himself from business meetings to attend his training session, saying he had to attend another meeting—only his wife and his PA knew that he was, in fact, going to a personal training session.

3. ROAM: An Entertraining Coaching Method

I created ROAM as a solution to the modern dilemma of compliance. Since 2000, I had been creating random programmes for the gym clients who had graduated from my three-phase programming, which corrected their injuries and posture through assessment, and stretching tight muscles and activating weak ones.

1. Co-ordinating the whole body with standing exercises emphasising the 6 Life movement patterns, moving in 3 dimensions, and using 8-12 repetition max sets.

2. Combining more than one life movement pattern emphasising movement slings, faster speeds, power, and agility.

Random programmes break from the linear progression of the health, fitness and performance phases while increasing an individual's movement periphery through unique combinations of exercises that activate new neuromuscular pathways of complexity, which keeps the body and brain guessing. This increases metabolic demand as well as enjoyment. Random programmes improve fitness, build muscle tone, and facilitate weight loss. Because they are not focused on one task in particular, they are not the best course of action to build big muscles or to peak for a sports competition.

Random programmes fit under the category I call *entertrainment*.

Entertrainment eradicates, or at least minimises, boredom in exercise. Random programmes are like a box of chocolates—you never know what you are going to get. Between 2000 and 2013, I wrote notebooks full of hundreds of unique training programme sessions for my clients.

In 2014, after growing bored of writing programmes for myself, I followed a Navy SEALs programme for three months. I would never have assigned these workouts for any of the three abovementioned phases, because, to my mind, the combinations lacked solid functional programme structure and order. Furthermore, they were gruelling—often taking me and my training partner an hour and a half to complete, but that was the fun of it. In terms of metabolic capacity, I was very fit, but I was not necessarily very strong or powerful in one area. The programme failed to address any of my weaknesses, although it did expose them.

What this programme has in common with CrossFit is that the workouts all have been given names. Names are entertaining; they serve as a benchmark that you can use to measure yourself against the rest of the world, as well as a means for going back and measuring your progress at another time.

I competed in three CrossFit opens, after which I realised I was fit and bodyweight-strong but not absolutely strong. Finding a skill lacking in my knowledge led me to seek strength training. I discovered Westside Barbell and followed their conjugate method, which moved away from pyramid-shaped periodisation into the conjugate system, which combines Maximum Effort Training and Dynamic Effort Training to increase strength and speed. It resembles a 1980s gymnastic programme in which you had to schedule six apparati into a training week, but they schedule bench press, squat and deadlift training into a week, all concentrating on a repetition max while using undulating volumes during the week and changes in two ranges, as well as one or two general physical preparation sessions.

ROAM combines all these systems with the added safety factor from corrective exercise. You'll progress through the life movement patterns, beginning with bodyweight flexibility first and working through to bodyweight ninja (a reasonable-difficulty bodyweight exercise), then to a barbell strength phase, using the accessory exercises from Westside and other modalities, and incorporating the natural method, which links each defence skill to a corresponding animal, and choosing the sport that expresses each life movement pattern. By the time you reach the performance stage, there are many crossovers of life movement patterns.

My goal as a movement coach is to increase my clients' range of active movement. This helps them to excel at life by working on their strengths and weaknesses, and it also helps to keep me engaged, so that I don't grow bored of counting endless tricep pushdowns. The variety of exercise is enjoyable, therefore encouraging people to engage with it regularly and consistently. This is where the health benefits come from.

ROAM is not a panacea; it is a device for general physical preparation for general fitness. It is suitable for beginners and the graduation provides a target. Those who are stressed out do not have to think so much about a balanced programme; they simply cycle between the animals. Elite athletes can cycle in an animal once a week in season, to keep fresh and break up sport-specific movements. During the off-season, cycling between all the animals for a certain period helps to counter pattern overuse.

ROAM is a system comprising of all other systems. As we move beyond the bodyweight phase, each ring represents many more exercises, because we add modalities of equipment in strength training. *(More on this in ROAM II: Function Meets Strength.)*

ROAM properties:

FASCIAL LINE	LIFE MOVE-MENT	FLEXI-BILITY	POSTURE	STABILITY	CRAWL	ANIMAL
Best fit	The key	Yoga Asana	Active	Yoga balance pose	Quadru-ped, infant develop-mental pattern	Five-element theory

26 ROAM: MOVEMENT AS MEDICINE

4. Goals, Benefits, and the Method

The goal is freedom or fluidity of movement

If the first step in a fitness journey is to start, the second is to make sure you avoid injury due to over-enthusiastic training in the two to three weeks after starting.

Elite athletes, concerned about remaining injury-free, invest a lot of training time into restoring freedom of motion to their joints and muscles and effectively utilising active recovery, and so should you.

The more sedentary or overweight you are, and the longer the gap between exercise, the more you need to restore your ability to move. Failure to do so will most likely result in an injury that will curtail any metabolic boosting (and fat loss or increase in fitness level).

A properly designed restoration programme helps you to identify potential problem areas. These problem areas are most often found at the intersection of tight and weak muscles and can be identified by looking at and assessing your individual posture.

When we stop using our bodies, we lose muscle tone and become flabby, and our systems become sluggish. Modern conveniences reduce our need to move. Most jobs nowadays are sedentary, requiring us to spend our days slouched over computers.

As our body adapts to what we habitually do, mankind is devolving into a three-toed sloth—slow-moving, sedentary for most of the day, and most likely overweight—primed for injury if required to fight or flee. The sloth is easy prey for predators. Leading a slothful life makes one prone to decay and disease, resulting in premature death.

Benefits of restoration exercise

The intensity of restoration exercise is at a low level—what I call window-shopping—pace. Any stretching or activity that increases circulation, involves movement of the whole body, isolates muscles or addresses out any imbalances from habitually doing one thing (or nothing at all) is considered restoration activity. In terms of percentage of maximum heart rate, it would be 60% or below, or a perceived exertion rate of easy to light.

The key is to first find something that you truly enjoy doing, so that you'll do it regularly and see some results that motivate you to keep exercising and to incorporate other types of exercise.

Some of the benefits of restoration exercise are:

- Health

- Longer life

- Positive and calm mindset

- Circulation of oxygen, blood and nutrients around the body

- Reactivation of isolated muscles

- Reintegration of muscles and joints to perform coordinated movements

- Freedom of motion in one joint or all joints in the body

- Postural alignment

Complementary to correcting your posture awareness is the restoration of flexibility and stability (mobility) to all joints and muscles. Yoga has an excellent system of mobility exercises and is suited to any ability.

Once mobility has been improved (bringing with it a degree of injury prevention) we can progress to metabolism-boosting strength, power, speed and agility fitness and performance training exercises.

Functional fitness pioneer Paul Chek noticed that most sports or activities are dominated by one or more combinations of *bend, pull, push, twist, squat, lunge* and *gait* movement patterns.

To restore health and function, improve fitness, and reach high performance, all of these movement patterns *must be included* in your weekly exercise programme.

This approach is the key to creating effective programming and exercise routines that are designed for the individual and is exemplified by my Five-Animal theme.

These whole movements can be regressed to smaller parts (usually ground-based), in order to isolate and stretch tight muscles or isolate and activate weak muscles. From there, we can then integrate these "smaller parts" until the whole movement can be performed with good technique.

These dominant movement patterns can be added together and combined in due course for further complexity, intensity and specificity in performance and play training. Different modalities such as the TRX Suspension Trainer, and other cables and free weights can be incorporated at any stage as teaching or progressions tools. By focusing on bodyweight exercises that can be done anywhere, I've removed the need to buy equipment and gym membership, which can be an obstacle to beginning a programme.

Unfortunately, most people do this the other way around, starting with complex movements that their bodies (and minds) may not be primed to perform safely and effectively. When we favour beginning with the "sexy", complex movements, which require greater coordination and muscle tension than we currently possess, we find that this is how we end up getting injured.

Mobility

After static postural training, we look to increase *mobility*, which can be defined as *range of motion with equal stability*. Chronic pain and overuse injuries occur when flexibility and stability are out of balance.

We can restore freedom of motion by correcting breathing mechanics, freeing fascial restrictions (I explain fascial lines in the next chapter), stretching muscles, and performing neuromuscular isolation and integration exercises to activate and stabilise muscles and joints.

The goal of mobility training is to remove the fear of pain from moving, and to encourage pain-free movement.

In whole-part-whole training, movement is both exercise and assessment. If the movement is restricted by muscle imbalances, it is broken down into manageable chunks to identify and isolate which muscles to stretch and which muscles to stabilise. Once we've corrected the muscle imbalances, the whole movement is performed and assessed again, then further broken down (in order to correct another aspect) and added to the movement repertoire or progressed in complexity.

In this example of whole-part-whole training, the life movement patterns are sequenced as five animal stretches. Each animal represents a life movement pattern. Each life movement pattern is assigned a corresponding full yoga asana. Each yoga asana is associated with a fascial line.

Whole

The full asana is a flexibility assessment: you either can or cannot do it. If you cannot do it, proceed to the part-stretch.

Part

The yoga asana is broken down into a series of individual stretches. After stretching the isolated muscle, re-do the full yoga asana, to test the efficacy of the part-stretch. If it results in greater range of motion of the full asana, or if it is easier or more fluid to perform, then you'll know that this part-stretch is beneficial for you.

This process will give you more freedom of motion in that movement pattern. You might cycle through all the life movement patterns during the week to broaden your range of active movement in all life movement patterns.

5. Life Movements and Five-Animal Fitness

The riddle of the wooden wheel

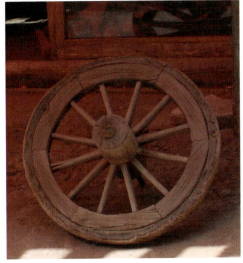

The word *yoga* derives from "yoke" or "union". This physical, mental and spiritual movement-based philosophy originated in India around 3,500 years ago. I took the photo shown above in Kashgar, China, in 2009. The wooden wheel comprises three main components:

1. Hub: the solid piece at the wheel's centre.

2. Spokes: the twelve segments join the hub to the rim, thereby providing structural integrity to the whole.

3. Tyre: the outer ring that makes contact with the road.

We know that this wheel will neither roll smoothly nor be able to support a heavy load if any of the above named three components are damaged or missing. The riddle: Which components pertain to the physical, mental and spiritual aspects of a human, respectively?

The main goal of yoga is to liberate us. We can take this to mean gaining freedom of physical movement, reaching optimal mental stress levels, and becoming spiritually enlightened. We can integrate body, mind and soul through physical practice and psychological intention.

Each yoga pose or asana has a targeted physical, mental and spiritual attribute. The mind sends the nerve stimulus via a nerve plexus to contract the muscles; the blood and breath circulates nutrients and oxygen; the muscle contraction moves specific organs, and glands and hormones are released and an attitude attained. Movement can be static or dynamic; fast or slow. Movement can be yoga or Qigong or baseball or tiddlywinks. All movement creates varying degrees of the same response. In yoga we can moderate the response, because each pose has a master pose that can be broken down into simpler subsets of the full pose, thereby allowing all levels of ability, condition and ambition to partake of its benefits.

Elemental Animals

After studying animals in nature, Qigong practitioners noticed behaviours, characteristics and traits that paralleled specific elemental properties, so they assigned a particular animal to each of the five elements.

The elemental animals vary from school to school, perhaps due to regional variances in climate, food source, habitat, and political intervention. As mentioned earlier, the Yellow Emperor forbade the use of the dragon as a symbol, as it was believed to possess mystical and magical powers that he did not want to share with the people.

Some teachers adhere to set forms they call the Five-Animal Frolics, which mimic the movement patterns of the animal; others believe that a less formal frolic, in which you just freestyle and channel your inner animal, can bring forth the same health benefits, especially when applied with the power of intention.

The YogaVinQi Code's five key animals and their corresponding elements:

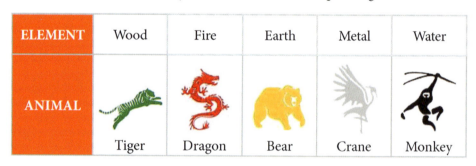

ELEMENT	Wood	Fire	Earth	Metal	Water
ANIMAL	Tiger	Dragon	Bear	Crane	Monkey

The allocation of the animals in the YogaVinQi Code is multi-faceted. At the first level, they mirror the Five-Element Theory (as presented by the CHEK Institute) matching life-movement patterns with animal-type movements, fascial and meridian lines, and yoga poses.

Life Movements and Five-Animal Fitness

I use five distinct animals to represent the dominant foundational patterns that are essential to our movement and mobility. The six life movements comprise: *squat, twist, bend, push, pull* and *lunge*.

Five-Animal Fitness can be applied to any modality, including bodyweight training, suspension training, kettlebells or free weights. The system is flexible and can be adapted to suit an individual's specific needs.

Each of the five animals—Tiger, Dragon, Bear, Crane and Monkey—exemplifies one or more of the fundamental movement patterns. This approach aims to restore range of active motion, improve posture and mobility, and facilitate progress to fitness and performance training.

There are roughly 1,350 yoga asanas. I have based *Movement as Medicine* and *The YogaVinQi Code* around five key asanas, according to these significant connections, cross-references and qualities:

- fascial lines
- infant developmental patterns
- life or functional movement patterns (squat, bend, lunge, twist, push, pull)
- animal movements
- mind-body connection
- the least amount of exercise to create the fastest and greatest return

For each of the key yoga asanas, I selected the animal whose primary characteristics represent its key movement patterns.

The five animals and their corresponding yoga asanas:

- Tiger: Modified Garland *(Utkatasana)*
- Bear: Deep Forward Bend *(Padangusthasana)*
- Crane: Warrior I *(Virabhadrasana I)*
- Dragon: Revolved Triangle *(Parivrtta Trikonasana)*
- Monkey: Warrior II *(Virabhadrasana II)*

These asanas are all standing poses and are called Big Bang stretches because of the freedom of movement they liberate. These full asanas represent how the body's movement has evolved over millennia. How each individual performs the poses provides valuable insights during assessment. If you cannot perform these poses or if you are reluctant to try, this can be viewed as a weakness (most likely induced by laziness or inertia). In order to restore freedom of movement, you must learn to perform these poses.

(Please note that for safety reasons, the following exercises are not recommended for the deconditioned or injured individual. If this applies to you, please turn to the appropriate movement chapter and perform stretches of a lower ability level. Gradually work your way up until you've developed enough flexibility, balance and confidence to attempt the full asana.)

34 ROAM: MOVEMENT AS MEDICINE

6. Identifying Your Power Animal

Power Animal

Your power animal is the animal related to the flexibility assessment that you do best. If you meet or exceed the standard shown in the photos, you likely possess the physical ability to do barbell strength training in that movement pattern with very low risk of injury.

Critical Animal

Your critical animal is the animal related to the flexibility assessment that you most struggle to do. If you are restricted in a life movement pattern you risk injury, because your brain and body compensate for your muscle imbalances by finding range of motion and stability elsewhere. The "elsewhere" joints and muscles will eventually protest with pain that, if you ignore it, will lead to other injuries and debilitation. It is critical in movement training to identify your areas of weakness and to strengthen them.

Five-Animal Flexibility Assessment

Perform all these poses as best as you comfortably can. In the appropriate column of the table, mark with a **Y** the ones you can do and mark with an **N** the ones you cannot do. Indicate the tight side by writing **R** or **L**. Rate the exercises according to which is your best (low priority) and which is your weakest (high priority). Essentially, you either can or cannot do them. For the exercises you cannot do, you will need to address these areas.

ASANA	YES/NO R/L RATING	CHAPTER
Overhead Squat		8
Forward Bend		9
Warrior I		10
Revolved Triangle		11
Warrior II		12

Chapters 8 through 12 will discuss your power and critical animals in greater depth, so you'll be able to prioritise the exercises to increase range of active movement and optimise the benefits.)

I have matched each of the five animals with a corresponding balance pose according to the following:

- A sense of flow, from one pose to the next

- Which fascial lines are activated or stretched

- A movement theme

- Key animal characteristics

- Elements and aspects of play

The five animals and their corresponding balance poses:

1. **Tiger:** Warrior III (Virabhadrasana III)

2. **Dragon:** Eagle (Garudasana)

3. **Bear:** Dancer (Natarajasana)

4. **Crane:** Handstand (Adho Mukha Vrksasana)

5. **Monkey:** Tree (Vrksasana")

Five-Animal Stability Assessment

These may or may not correspond to the flexibility assessment. In the instance that they do correspond, you have identified a higher priority. (If you are concerned that any of these balances are too difficult or may result in injury, please refrain from doing them. Simply mark them with an **X** to indicate a critical area that needs to be addressed.)

Five-Animal Stability Assessment

ASANA	RESULTS	CHAPTER
Warrior III		8
Eagle		9
Dancer		10
Handstand		11
Tree		12

In the following chapters, I will discuss in greater detail each of the five animals and their respective key asanas and balance poses. My iPhone App *5-Animal Mobility* demonstrates all of these poses, movements and balances via high-quality photographs and video clips, and provides detailed instructions for how to perform them in a safe and effective manner.

The full yoga asanas, balance poses, and crawl patterns of the five animals serve to lengthen, activate and integrate all the fascial lines, thereby safely increasing your range of active movement. Daily practice of the five animal exercises helps to prevent overuse injuries. If you specialise in a particular sport and have a gradual-onset injury, restoration may be enhanced by performing the animal exercises that most closely mimic this sport.

In yoga, exercise is performed in accordance with the rhythm of the breath. A slow breathing pace helps to decelerate the metabolism and has a calming effect. A rapid breathing pace accelerates the metabolism and has an energising effect. It is best to perform restoration exercises at a slow pace and to perform fitness training at a fast pace.

40 ROAM: MOVEMENT AS MEDICINE

7. The Journey of Man

Movement is medicine. Movement helps us adapt to our environment and its dangers by developing our reflexes and urges. The problem with modern life is that we are regressing and devolving in our movement habits. We've already discussed how modern life renders movement less necessary, thereby engendering slothful and sedentary lifestyles. But even those of us who are athletic and active are at risk. As we specialise in a particular sport, we accumulate pattern-overload postures and muscle imbalances that may lead to injury. Being inactive and injured lowers our energy levels, increases our fat percentage and makes us apathetic and depressed.

Charles Darwin said that only organisms that adapt to fit their environment can survive and thrive. Man's ability to walk, run, jump and play is a hybrid of movement patterns gained during the evolution from single-celled amoeba to homo sapien.

Billions of years ago, life started as a single-cell organism with a mouth and a digestive system. It survived by waiting for food to flow into its mouth. Over time, food became scarce, and we became food for others. These two threats—starvation and predators—provoked evolution's first step, of growing external vila that we could flutter in order to move, so that we could hunt for food and escape predators. This pattern was repeated countless times until we reached our present state and follows roughly this outline:

The vila gradually evolved into the five-limbed starfish with its mouth situated where the umbilicus is now. The starfish developed fins and evolved into the fish, its head and tail joined by a lateral moving spine. Its fins developed into arms and legs, and it became the land-based reptile.

This progression, from passive stationary creature to dynamic hunter creature, requires the central nervous system to coordinate thought with movement: the drive to eat and to be safe is physically expressed. The central nervous system is an extension of our brain and it governs all our actions.

The nervous system has a central control centre called the brain. Two nerve branches (autonomic nervous system) carry specific messages from the brain to different parts of the body and back again. The sympathetic branch is responsible for movement (fight or flight) and the parasympathetic branch is responsible for recovery (rest and digestion). The mindmap below illustrates the functions of these polar complementary systems.

Autonomic Nervous System

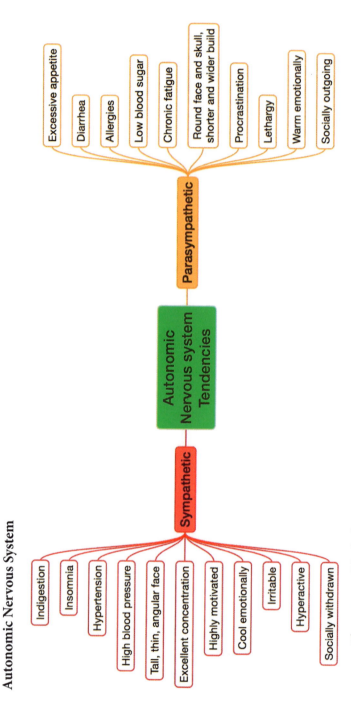

The systems of the body operate in a two-way relationship. One system drives us to catch food and a parallel system helps us to recover from the hunt and digest the food. When we are hungry we hunt; when we are satiated we rest. These systems are complementary and help to balance life. Any imbalance between these systems will lead to a decrease in health.

Nerve Plexus

The nervous system's superhighway comprises intersections of nerve bundles called plexus. There are seven major nerve plexus in the body. Each nerve plexus has an endocrine gland that performs a specific function in the body. Each gland has two hormones: one for helping to switch the function on, and another for helping to switch it off.

The mind map below lists the glands and their functions and dominant hormones.

Nerve Plexus, endocrine gland, hormones and function

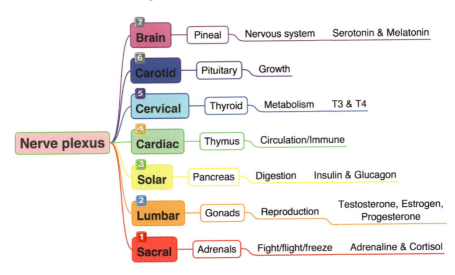

This complex system of systems took a long time to evolve. We will now break down the development of the central nervous system into evolutionary stages and three main steps.

Triune brain

In *The Triune Brain in Evolution*, author and neuroscientist Paul D. Maclean provides a good model for understanding what Darwin meant when he said: "The one most responsive to change survives."

Essentially, we have developed three parts to our current brain: reptilian, mammalian, and paleomammalian. Each part of the brain is responsible for satisfying our needs and wants, which are governed by certain drives and reflexes, and are presented in Maslow's Hierarchy of Needs. Evolution follows circumstance and the value we place on these wants and needs.

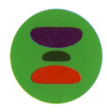

This icon represents the three brains and their respective values.

Red: Reptilian brain and survival/movement, sustenance, and procreation.

Green: Mammalian brain and emotions, love, and social affiliation.

Violet: Neocortical (human) brain and communication, creativity, and spirituality.

These values are stacked in a delicate balance with the "I" survival needs of safety, food and procreation providing the base, The "we" emotional needs are in the middle and provide the spiritual bridge to the altruistic "all" thinking and self-actualisation drivers.

The human brain is so intelligent it can override symptoms of pain, fatigue and emotion for long periods of time to satisfy social status. About fifteen years of ignoring symptoms is how long it takes to manifest a serious disease. As modern job specialisation requires us to use our brains more, we use our bodies less. As the body falls into disrepair and sloth, mental pressure saps our motivation and engenders a negative mindset.

1. Reptilian brain

Our first brain, developed at the lizard stage, is called the reptilian brain. The reptilian brain is the instinctive selfish brain concerned only with "I" and the three needs needed to survive and thrive:

1. Safety: fight or flight or freeze (survive)
2. Sustenance: food and water (survive)
3. Sex: the desire to continue the species (thrive)

These three needs are not taught. The reptilian brain stores reflexes, instincts and responses and uses the adrenals glands to help control them. As such, the walnut-sized adrenal glands sitting on top of our kidneys influence the musculoskeletal system, digestion, and the production of sex hormones. In newborns, we see reflexes to grasp and suck a nipple, to wiggle to search for food, to cry when it can't find any food, and to sleep when satiated, and to grow.

All the movements we perform as babies (wiggling, sucking toes, turning over and crawling) turn on reflexes that switch on and release hormones and neurotransmitters in the brain, promoting growth and development of the newborn's senses, movement, and understanding of the world.

There are several infant developmental patterns performed by the baby whilst exploring its environment. The wiggle and the inchworm are two such movements performed when reaching for a rattle or searching for a toy. The wiggle is an example of the reptilian lateral moving spine (Dragon, Twist), and the inchworm of the mammalian spine (Tiger, Squat).

All of these infant developmental patterns are performed into adulthood and they continue to activate the plexus, glands, hormones and functions.

2.Mammalian brain

The next jump on the evolutionary ladder is from cold-blooded reptile to warm-blooded mammal. The spine moves on a vertical articulation. Mammalian crawling patterns stimulate the integration of left and right brain hemispheres.

Emotions start in the mammalian brain

The mammalian brain is the "we" brain and is concerned with community, the fourth need of love and social affiliation demonstrated by the parental bond and the tendency for mammals to congregate in herds.

The mammalian brain recognises the wants and needs of love and emotion (which we will discuss in greater depth in later chapters).

If a baby does not crawl, this may indicate coordination and learning difficulties in later life. Some examples being:

- dyspraxia (loss of balance seen as clumsiness)

- dyslexia (reading and writing problems)

- underdeveloped coordination

- autism and attention deficit disorders

Fortunately, we can retrain neuromuscular pathways by performing developmental crawling patterns and other Western and Eastern movement systems.

3. Neocortical (human) brain

Our third and final brain is our most powerful one. We use the neocortical brain to:

1. communicate in complex languages
2. invent labour-saving tools
3. form the collective consciousness known as culture

The triune brain is a model that serves the purpose of describing motivation to move. It helps us understand Darwinian theory. The illustration below gives a rough overview of the evolution of man over millions of years and serves as a model of movement that simplifies and unifies the YogaVinQi Code.

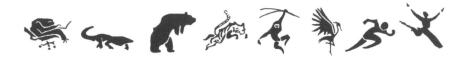

These animals—Sloth, Dragon, Bear, Tiger, Monkey, Crane—represent the infant developmental pattern followed by human babies from birth to standing up. The Running Man signifies the human gait of walking and running; the Leaping Man symbolises the human capacity to combine all of the movement patterns at once.

Every icon except the sloth represents:

- a dominant triune brain
- nerve plexus
- gland and its hormones and function
- everyday movement pattern
- best-fit dominant fascial line

8. Vitruvian Man and Fascial Lines

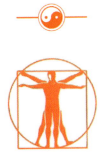

Leonardo da Vinci believed that the ideal man would fit cleanly into a circle, as depicted in his famous drawing, *The Vitruvian Man*.

Da Vinci based this illustration on the ideal human proportions posited by the Roman architect Vitruvius. Da Vinci noted that:

- The length of the outspread arms is equal to the height of a man.
- The face from the chin to the lowest roots of the hair can be split into three equal parts, known as the rule of thirds. When you look at many people in society today, you will notice that their faces follow the rule of thirds.
- The combination of arm and leg positions creates 16 different poses.
- The drawing combines art and science in its creation.
- The drawing is used as a symbol of symmetry of the body and of the universe as a whole.

The most common understanding of the Vitruvian Man from a Western scientific viewpoint is as a symbol of balance and symmetry of the body. What is less commonly appreciated is that the Vitruvian Man also represents the balance of the mind and the spirit. It is difficult to balance one without balancing the other. Consequently, when one part is out of balance, both are out of balance, resulting in a decrease in health, fitness and performance.

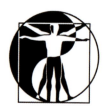

The body-mind-spirit field is a massive, complex and unrecognised in the fitness industry. To keep things focused on movement I have omitted a section showing the parallels of Eastern metaphysical wisdom and Western neuroscience called "The YogaVinQi Code" and inserted into my upcoming book "Sort your Life out". "Sort your life out" uses the LIFE cycle wheel as an assessment tool to addressing work-life and vitality imbalances. The YogaVinQi Code combines the physical-mental-emotional and spiritual aspects of yoga, vitruvian man and the five element theory of Qi, with the four solutions - Lifestyle, Intention, Food and Exercise. Used in "Sort you life out" they can provide further diagnostic themes and avenues of solutions to you work-life-vitality imbalances.

Fascial Lines

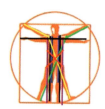

What is fascia?

Fascia is a band of connective tissue joining together the muscles. Much like the skin of a sausage, it surrounds individual muscles and links muscles together in what we call muscle chains or fascial lines. The two types of muscle chains are:

- the flexor chain produces forward bending by contracting most of the muscles in the front of the body

- the extensor chain extends the body back up again

Each muscle chain has specific functions. The performance of complex movements requires simultaneously engaging a combination of them. Fascial lines are spokes in the wheel to create movement. Together they form the basis of the Western viewpoint of movement as seen in *The Vitruvian Man*.

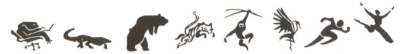

ANIMAL	SLOTH	DRAGON	BEAR	TIGER	MONKEY	CRANE	MAN	PLAY
Dominant Fascial Lines		Spiral	Superficial back	Superficial front, Deep front	Back arm lines, lateral	Front arm lines	Functional lines, lateral	All
Movement		Twist	Bend	Squat	Pull, (Lunge)	Push (lunge)	Walk, run	Leap
Crawl Pattern		Offset Press Up crawl, wiggle	Ipsi lateral	Contra lateral, inchworm	Lateral hop	Single leg hip hinge		

Much research has been conducted recently on fascia to gain a better understanding of how it works and the role it plays in mobility, movement and restoration of function.

Manual therapist Thomas Myers has been at the forefront of illustrating the role of fascia in the body through his book *Anatomy Trains: Myofascial Meridians for Manual and Movement Therapists*.

Table 1 simplifies Myers' fascial lines and gives their locations and the basic movements they produce. While it may appear overwhelming to the layman, I've included it only to provide some background understanding and will break down these fascial lines into five key yoga asanas and their families.

Fascial lines are an adaptation of necessity and show the evolution of the journey of man. In the following pages, I will use the Five-Animal Method to express these concepts in one unifying approach.

Table 1: Fascial lines, location and movement

FASCIAL LINE	LOCATION	MOVEMENT
Superficial back	Back, length of whole body	Backwards
Superficial front	Front, length of whole body	Forwards
Lateral	Side, length of whole body	Sideways
Spiral	Front abdominal, lateral legs, back legs, deep back spine	Twisting
Superficial front arm	Front forearm	Bend arm
Deep front arm	Front upper arm	Bend arm
Superficial back arm	Back forearm	Straighten arm
Deep back arm	Back upper arm	Straighten arm
Back Functional	Back, butt, quads	Pull/twist backwards
Front functional	Chest, abdominals, groin	Push/twist forwards
Ipsilateral Functional	Side trunk and outside thigh	Side bend
Deep front	Front, deep, length of body	Bending forwards and breathing

Meridian Lines

Meridian lines closely follow fascial lines. Qi flows through the channels just as water flows through streams and rivers. In man, there are twelve primary meridians; these are bilateral and symmetrical. The channels can be identified according to the Yin or Yang organ to which they are connected, and by the limbs in which the channels originate or end.

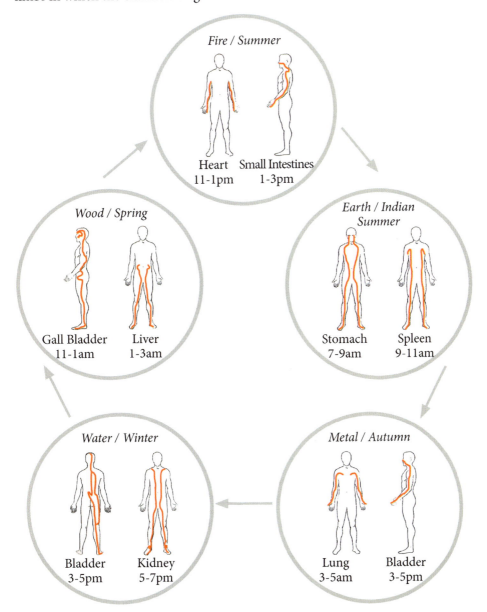

Note: I have only included the 10 main meridians in this five element model.

52   ROAM: MOVEMENT AS MEDICINE

9. Restoration Begins With Posture

The Running Man	Functional and Lateral Lines
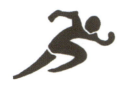	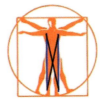

The Running Man is allocated to walking and running, and to the "standing still" movement pattern that we call standing posture. The Running Man represents man's ability to stand upright and walk out of the protection of the jungle and combines all of the other animals' locomotion patterns.

Running is an upright contralateral pattern. When one foot strikes the ground, the opposite arm extends forward and the back functional line is activated (this overlaps strongly with the Monkey). As the toe of the opposite leg pushes off, the opposite arm is tensed. This is called the front functional line (overlaps with the Crane). When the body is vertically balanced, the lateral line is active (as with any single leg balances).

All fascial lines contribute to all movement. All life movements have one or two lines that are predominant. When we are injured, fascial lines help us to locate and isolate which individual muscles to treat.

The Running Man represents the human gait at its highest order. Human gait is upright walking, running and sprinting. Before we can run, we first need to crawl. This is what we learn from the other animals, and this leads to sprinting and leaping.

Movement begins and ends with good posture. Before we can crawl, we need to restore good posture.

Restoration begins with correct posture

When restarting exercise after a long layoff, we must start by correcting the posture. Stacking the body so that a line bisects the ankle bone, the centre of the knee, the hip, the shoulder, and the centre of the ear lobe constitutes correct posture, as shown in Posture A in the diagram below.

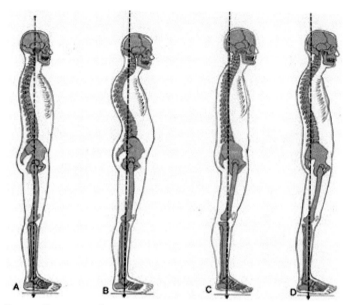

Source: *Posture and Function (Florence Kendall)*

Postures B, C and *D* all depict typical patterns of weak and tight muscles pulling the skeleton out of alignment. The restriction of the range of motion, combined with too great a volume of work (particularly when moving a heavy load or moving a large distance at high speed), will eventually result in injury, even for elite athletes.

In my many years' experience of measuring the posture curves and flexibility imbalances of individuals, I have seen normal posture (A) and flat-back posture (C) each in about 2% of all cases, with the remaining 96% split evenly between the other two types. A person with Kyphosis-Lordosis (or KL) posture (B) is prone to instability injuries because of the exaggerated curves. A person with sway-back (or SB) posture (D) is prone to disc injuries because bending forward with rotation places increased pressure on the discs.

The major difference between the sway-back and KL postures can be seen at the lumbar spine and pelvis, where the muscle imbalances are opposite, which means that the same exercise programme will reduce imbalances in one but increase it in the other. For this reason, it is essential that restoration exercise programmes address the unique condition of each individual.

Warm-up instructions

A warm-up is designed to elevate the temperature of the body to make it more pliable for movement. Rehearsing the movements you're about to perform helps to switch on the brain and activate the nerve system that carries messages from the brain to the muscular system. A dynamic warm-up is identified by fluid, continuous and easy movements performed at about 60% of capacity.

(For a thorough and comprehensive dynamic warm-up routine, check out my free iPhone app *Bodyweight Ninja*, which offers a dynamic warm-up routine for sports and physical activity. Performed at a faster pace, this routine is designed to raise your body temperature, get your blood flowing, activate the nervous system, increase your range of motion, and help get your mind into the zone. When the sequence is performed at a slow and easy breathing pace, you will find it to be an effective cool-down for your muscles, as well as helping to calm your mind and the rest of the nervous system.)

Static Stretching instructions

The purpose of a static stretch is to lengthen the muscles to improve joint range of motion and movement fluidity. Go into and out of all stretches gently and gradually, and, if possible, perform them as you exhale the breath. Muscles have a protective mechanism known as the stretch reflex, which offers strong resistance to help prevent overstretching and injury. When you move gently into a stretch, the threat of injury is lower than if you move rapidly into a stretch, so the stretch reflex will not be as quickly activated.

Let's say that on a scale of 0 through 10, 0 signifies asleep and 10 severe pain. You will start feeling a stretch in the range of about 4 to 6; and at about 8 the stretch reflex will become active and resist further extension. In my opinion the optimal stretch sensation lies at around 7, and that's where you'll get the best return for your efforts. In order to override the stretch reflex, the brain has to send a message indicating that the current range of motion is safe, and it takes between six and ten seconds for this message to reach the stretch reflex. By the time it releases and allows you to push further, the 7 may have decreased to a 5 or 6. A stretch that has been held for 60 seconds may have up to 6 releases, thus significantly improving range of motion.

To enhance the stretch reflex mechanism:

- Time your exhale with the release, as exhalation relaxes the body and mind

- Consciously relax the stretched muscle (requires practice)

- Keep the stretch tension at a constant 7-10

- Hold the stretch for as long as you are making gains—this could be shorter or longer than a minute

Three posture points and three posture exercises

The postural restoration exercises Wall Lean, Scarecrow and Standing Cobra can be performed by anyone with KL posture. What is almost universal in posture dysfunction is forward-head posture, where the ear is forward of the plumb line and the increase curve of the upper back (thoracic spine). With the increasing popularity of smartphones, these postural faults are only going to get worse. I believe these three postural restoration exercises are integral to maintaining and improving your quality of life.

1. Stand tall, with ears, shoulders, hips, knees and ankles in alignment.
2. Distribute your weight evenly on both feet.
3. Squeeze your shoulder blades together and slightly draw in your abdominals.

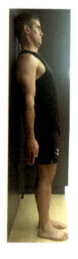

1. Wall Lean

  i. Stand with your back against a wall and then move both your feet one shoe length away from the wall.
  ii. Keeping your head against the wall, tuck in your chin until your cheekbone is in line with your collarbone.
  iii. Move your backside, spine and shoulders away from the wall. (The back of your head is the only point that should be in contact with the wall.)
  iv. Hold for 10 seconds, then place your backside against the wall in a resting position for 10 seconds.

(Repeat 10 times)

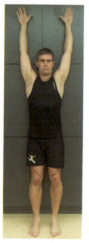

2. Scarecrow

  i. Stand with your back against a wall and then move both your feet one shoe length away from the wall.
  ii. Bend your elbows to 90 degrees to assume a scarecrow pose with elbows and backs of hands touching the wall.
  iii. Tuck in your backside, so that your lower back is in contact with the wall.
  iv. Slide your elbows up the wall until just before they break contact with the wall, and then slide back down to the starting position.

(Slowly repeat 15 times)

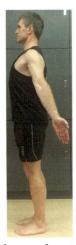

3. Standing Cobra

i. Stand with correct posture (chin tucked in, and ears, shoulders, hips and knees in alignment).

ii. Inhale.

iii. Lift chest up to reverse upper back curve.

iv. Turn arms and hands outwards. Keep shoulders down and away from ears.

v. Squeeze shoulder blades together.

vi. When you need to exhale, return to your resting position.

(Repeat for 2 - 5 minutes)

After performing these three exercises for thirty consecutive days, you will feel better and look taller and slimmer, and you will have greater confidence and poise. After thirty days, your standing posture will more closely resemble the standing prone cobra.

> "Proper posture enables graceful movement, relaxes the mind, calms the heart and brings confidence to your life force."

Neuroscience studies have shown a measurable increase of testosterone and decrease of cortisol in subjects who hold power postures for two or more minutes. Ancient medical systems including yoga and Qigong have been aware of the effect of body posture since 3,500 years ago. That's why they developed systems of movement comprising asanas to improve circulation, muscle tone, and mindset, to unify the body and stimulate the healing of joints, muscles, organs, glands, emotions, and disease.

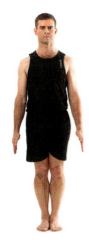

In yoga, correct posture, as described earlier and illustrated in the diagram **Posture A**, is called Mountain Pose (or *Tadasana*). In Qigong it is called Wuji. Yogis and TCM practitioners alike talk about the "rod of light" or Taiji that runs from the perineum to the crown of the head, aligning the seven main yoga chakras or the three Chinese Dantians.

Tadasana

The Tadasana pose is performed at the beginning of most yoga and Qigong practices because it helps start the process of unifying the body, mind and spirit. Yoga has around fifteen

Tadasana teaching cues and in the Dao Yin medical Qigong postural training, there are eighteen rules of postural alignment.

In essence, good posture requires a neutral spine, with the centre of the ears, shoulders, hips, knees and ankles in alignment. This is the most efficient position to move in and from. Life's pressures pull or push us out of this posture, creating muscle imbalances that cause dysfunction and make it difficult for us to move.

By stretching an isolated muscle, you can identify a weak link in the fascial line and remove restrictions above and below a joint, in order to free up an entire movement pattern. Stretching and stability exercises increase your mobility and movement. Several other specific posture exercises help keep your body in good alignment.

The Leaping Man

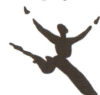

All Fascial Lines

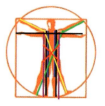

The Leaping Man is the final stage of the YogaVinQi Code and represents performance and play. The Leaping Man is the combination of all fascial lines and all the range of active movement that this equation allows.

Watch the victor at a sporting event or any person experiencing triumph and you will notice that they throw their arms up in the air. Why? Blind people also throw their arms in the air when experiencing joy, which proves that it is innate, instinctual behaviour rather than something they have observed and learned. We throw our arms up in the air when experiencing elation because it feels good. It feels good, because it raises testosterone and lowers the stress hormone cortisol.

The Leaping Man is a symbol of jumping for joy. This can be an internal sense or external expression of ecstasy from triumphing over others in sport, or simply from the pleasure of the experience, the opportunity, the freedom to create any movement that makes you *feel* good.

In this modern world we need not catch our food nor run away from predators on a daily basis. We can choose to express our spirit and joy of life through movement. The Leaping Man represents the freedom to choose how to experience and express joy. The experience does not need to result in a gold medal, nor does it require people to watch it. The expression (movement) is its own reward.

Your goal is to finding your own Leaping Man. You can achieve this through uninhibited play, as seen in a children's playground, or an unstructured warm-up activity before sports.

To help you build your Leaping Man, we separate its accumulation into distinct moving parts and order them according to the generation cycle of Five-Element Theory. Squatting, twisting, bending, pushing and pulling. (Lunging is included within the pulling and pushing patterns). Any movement coordinating opposite arms and legs uses the functional back and front lines.

The following chapters will explain each life movement pattern and break it down into components, in order to find the weak link and restore its proper contribution to the whole movement pattern.

10. Squat Like a Tiger

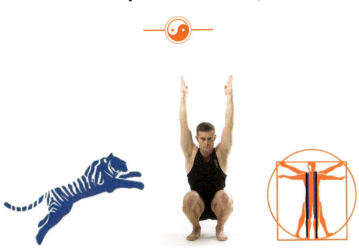

ROAM properties: Squat

FASCIAL LINE	LIFE MOVEMENT	FLEXIBILITY	POSTURE	STABILITY	CRAWL	ANIMAL
Superficial front, Deep front	Squat	Overhead Squat	Scarecrow, Plank	Warrior III	Contralateral	Tiger

The squat is the movement we perform most often in life. We squat to get out of bed; to sit on and rise from the toilet; to sit on a chair at mealtimes; to ride in the car, bus or train during our commute; and at the desk in the workplace. Olympic lifters squat in both the clean and jerk, and the snatch. Power lifters have one event called the squat. Basketball, volleyball, and all other jumping sports have the squat as the foundational or prerequisite movement for performance. All human beings are able to do a full squat as a transition movement from crawling to standing in their first year of life. When I ask the majority of Western people to squat, I am usually met with groans and moans, or mirth and embarrassment about their lack of range of motion. Ask the same question to Asian, African, South American and some European people, and they can squat right down, "arse to grass", without any problem. The difference stems not from genetics (nature) but from their environment (nurture). Many cultures do not use seating apparati as much as Western cultures do, particularly when going to the bathroom.

Having a full range of motion in your squat decreases your chances of getting injured and increases your performance ability when doing any bodyweight squat-related movement. (However, caution must be applied with additional loads, such as barbells, because a rounded back puts significant pressure on the intervertebral discs and can lead to debilitating back pain.) Squats can help rehabilitate the back, because increasing the muscle tone and strength of the thighs and buttocks, in conjunction with active abdominals, takes the load off the back. Let's further explore these relationships.

Fascial lines

The superficial and deep front lines are allocated to the squat. Within the stretch series, the allocation of the frontal lines is not as apparent as the other movement patterns and fascial lines. The squat in my opinion is the best fit for the frontal lines because of the engagement of the thighs and the abdominals. Performing one or all of the squat stretches (listed below) for thirty days will return significant gains in your squat flexibility.

(Please note: The physical relationship of animals, movements and fascial lines may not match up completely in a Western body view. Allocations will be reconciled and explained in full when we add the Eastern mind and spirit view in *The YogaVinQi Code*.)

Yoga flexibility pose, assessment and standard

The yoga asana for the squat movement is a deep squat, combining the Chair Pose (*Utkatasana*) and the Garland. This deep squat assessment provides us with feedback to the health and mobility of your ankles, knees, hips and lumbar spine. The overhead squat provides feedback about thoracic spine mobility.

- In powerlifting, a squat is deemed deep enough when the fold of the hips is parallel with, or lower than, the crease of the knee.

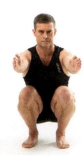

Squat Test 1: Lower body

- Keeping your arms below the level of your shoulders, squat down.

- A pass is being able to get the hips below the level of the knees. Heels must be flat on the ground, and feet and hips must be symmetrical.

- A pass here indicates that your ankles, knees, hips and lumbar spine have good mobility and you can move to Squat Test 2.

- If you cannot reach standard, this is an indication that the Tiger is your Critical Animal, and you need to address the deficit in range of active movement by doing all of the squat stretches.

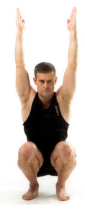

Squat Test 2: Lower and upper body

- This test is performed with your arms extended straight above your head and level with your ears the whole time.

- If you cannot perform this squat, this indicates that your thoracic spine and latissimus dorsi are tight and you need to concentrate on these areas.

- If you can perform this squat, you can consider the Tiger to be your Power Animal.

SQUAT DYNAMIC WARM-UP	REPS OR TIME
Air Squat	3 reps at moderate pace
Squat forward	3 reps at moderate pace
Overhead Squat	3 reps at moderate pace

Test, stretch, and retest

After your warm-up, perform the yoga flexibility pose to set a benchmark for the day, perform one stretch, and then retest. Cycle through the stretch series and determine which stretch is most effective for your body. This is the one you should concentrate on when you are short of time.

Stretch series: Squat/Tiger

SQUAT STRETCH SERIES	REPS OR TIME
Soleus Stretch	1 min each leg
Lats Stretch	1 min each side
Spine Extension 1	2-3 mins at each segment max 3 segments

ROAM: MOVEMENT AS MEDICINE 65

SQUAT STRETCH SERIES	REPS OR TIME
Hamstring Stretch 1	1 min each leg
Quad Stretch	1 min each leg
Hindi Squat	16 breaths

Movement and posture activation exercises for the Tiger

After stretching has created a new range of motion for the day, we can assimilate that extra flexibility and fluidity into the body with resistance exercises. In some cases, range of motion will not improve unless the muscles surrounding a joint have been activated or made to feel secure. The following exercises are aimed to do this at a health level of intensity and complexity. (If any of these movements should cause pain after the flexibility portion, please seek professional advice for some hands-on treatment.)

Range of active movement exercises for the Tiger

SQUAT MOBILITY	REPS OR TIME	TEMPO	ROUNDS
Plank	5	5 sec hold 5 second rest	1-3
Tiger Crawl	5 each side	Slow and controlled	1-3
Dynamic squats	10	3 seconds down and 3 seconds up	1-3
Scarecrow	15	Slow, sliding elbows up and down wall.	1-3
Plank Knee tucks	10	1 second in and 1 second out	1-3

One round comprises all five exercises. If you feel that one round is not stimulating enough, perform another one or two rounds, taking as much rest as you need between rounds.

As a matter of interest, perform your initial flexibility test to see if the muscle activation has improved your range of active movement.

Movement stability and yoga balance

The Warrior III single leg balance pose (Virabhadrasana III) requires the abdominals of the frontal line to be active. Aesthetically speaking, Warrior III is reminiscent of a tiger leaping through the air to pounce on its prey.

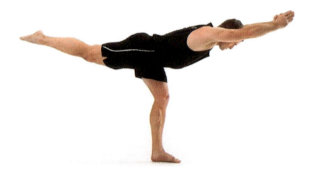

Perform the pose for 5 breaths on each leg, up to three times for each leg.

After following this programme for four to six weeks, you will see a significant improvement in your squat range of movement and stability.

Why is the Tiger the Power Animal of the squat?

The tiger stalks its prey in the jungle and uses its powerful back legs to close the kill distance with a massive pounce. This movement closely resembles the squat. An exercise that engages the frontal lines is called the Plank (Chaturanga in yoga). The Tiger crawling pattern is a contralateral moving plank, in which opposite arms and legs move at the same time. Crawling patterns are quadrupedal (four-footed) movements and are used extensively in recreational gymnastics, parkour, and military obstacle courses.

11. Twist Like a Dragon

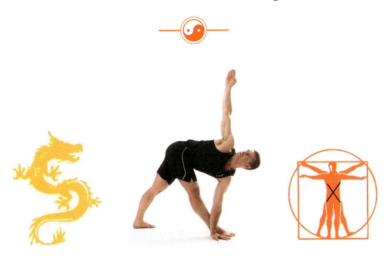

ROAM properties: Twist

FASCIAL LINE	LIFE MOVEMENT	FLEXIBILITY	POSTURE	STABILITY	CRAWL	ANIMAL
Spiral	Twist	Revolved Triangle	Horse stance Dynamic	Eagle	Crawling asymmetrical push-up	Dragon

The spine rotates and side-bends through the twisting of individual vertebrae. When we walk, each arm swings forward in time with the opposite leg, allowing the shoulders to counter-rotate the pelvis. Eighty-five percent of the core muscles orientate diagonally, facilitating twisting activities, such as playing racquet sports, throwing a ball or a stone, or resisting rotation when pushing or pulling open a door.

This twisting movement pattern uses the most stretches, and mobilises the most movement, involving many joints and muscles. Hamstrings play a large role in restricting the lumbar spine; and lats and pecs in restricting the rotation and extension of the thoracic spine.

Benefits

If you play any sport that requires you to swing a racquet, club or stick, then development of this pose will help prevent injury and enhance performance. As we age, the spine's ability to rotate decreases, and this can lead to muscle strain or other injuries. Keeping an active range of movement in the twist pattern helps prevents injury. Any twisting movement in the abdominal region also massages the organs of digestion.

Fascial lines

The dominant fascial lines associated with the lateral bending and twisting of the spine are the lateral line, spiral line, and functional lateral line.

Yoga flexibility pose assessment and standard

The Dragon asana and life movement is the Revolved Triangle (*Parivrtta Trikonasana*) and the twist. The Revolved Triangle asana twists the spine, stretches the front-leg hamstring group, and strengthens the legs and the core.

The test procedure is simple: you either can or cannot do it to standard. If you cannot, this indicates that you require a period of restoration of range and stability of movement to regain function.

The Revolved Triangle is an advanced and complex yoga pose that involves the spine, the hips, the groin, and the hamstrings. Chances are that one or more of these muscles will limit your performance, so if you are unsure, attempt it close to a solid wall or perform the pose at an easier level by bringing your hand off the floor and resting it high on your leg.

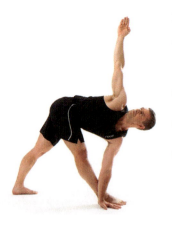

Revolved Triangle Standard

- Back leg turned out to 45 degrees; front leg straight forward
- Both legs straight
- Keeping a flat back, rotate spine to opposite leg
- With one hand on the floor and the other vertical, look upwards at the vertical arm

Stretch series for the Dragon

TWIST STRETCH SERIES	REPS OR TIME
Revolved triangle	5 breaths
Lying rotation	1 min each side
Supine Glutes	1 min each side
Hamstring (cross body)	1 min each side

TWIST STRETCH SERIES	REPS OR TIME
Pec Minor Stretch	1 min each side
Thread the needle dynamic	15 reps each side
Seated needle stretch	1 min each side
Frog-dynamic	15 reps

TWIST STRETCH SERIES	REPS OR TIME
Frog-static	1 min each side
Seated Rotation	1 min each side
Triangle	16 breaths

Movement and posture activation exercises for the Dragon

The Dragon crawling pattern is another variation of the plank and is the closest to the Four-Limbed Staff Pose or low plank (*Chaturanga Dandasana*). The crawl moves forward after a push-up with the arms in an offset position.

Range of active movement exercises for the Dragon

TWIST MOBILITY	REPS OR TIME	TEMPO	ROUNDS
Novice dragon crawls	x 10 forward and back	2 sec down and 2 sec up	1-3
Novice offset push ups	x5 each side	2 sec down and 2 sec up	1-3
Mountain climbers	x 10 ea	1 sec forward and 1 sec back	1-3
Russian twist	8-12 ea	2 sec down and 2 sec up	1-3

TWIST MOBILITY	REPS OR TIME	TEMPO	ROUNDS
Static horse	10 reps each alternating side	10 sec hold each side	1-3
Dynamic horse	10	Inhale to extend, exhale to bend	1-3

Perform 1-3 rounds (a round is a completion of all 6 exercises).

Movement stability and yoga balance

The Eagle pose (*Garudasana*) is the single leg balance pose for the twist pattern. It activates and stretches the spiral line and arm lines of the muscles used to stabilise the Komodo Dragon push-up/crawl movement.

- The single leg balance for the Dragon involves twisting/coiling the arms and legs across each other

- Hold the balance for 5 breaths each side

- (Repeat 1-3 times)

After following this programme for four to six weeks, you'll see a significant improvement in your twisting range of movement and stability.

Why is the Dragon the Power Animal of the twist?

The sideways articulation of the spine is seen in the movements of the shark, lizard, crocodile, and Komodo dragon.

10. Bend Like a Bear

The Bear   Superficial back line (as viewed from the front)

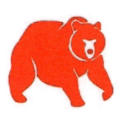
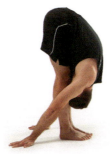
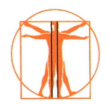

ROAM properties: Bend

FASCIAL LINE	LIFE MOVE-MENT	FLEXI-BILITY	POSTURE	STABILITY	CRAWL	ANIMAL
Superficial back	Bend	Forward bend	Locust	Dancer	Ipsilateral	Bear

The difference between the bend and the squat is that the bend hinges at the hips and involves only a relatively slight bending of the knees. The lifting occurs mostly from the cantilever-type arrangement of the hamstrings and the butt and lower back muscles.

Benefits

The bend is related to the squat in the sense that we use this life movement when we pick things up off the floor. We bend to pick up groceries or babies. We bend to pick up light or heavy objects.

Fascial lines

The fascial line most responsible for this back extension is the superficial back line.

Yoga flexibility pose assessment and standard

The Bear's asana and life movement is the deep forward bend (*Padangusthasana*). This asana lengthens the hamstrings and lower back muscles that allow safe lifting posture in the bend movement patterns. The deadlift is the most common bend pattern in weightlifting and progresses to the Olympic-lifting overhead snatch.

The test procedure is simple: you either can or cannot do it to standard. If you cannot, this indicates that you require a period of restoration of range and stability of movement to regain function.

The forward bend involves the calves, hamstrings, and back spinal muscles and indicates your risk of a disc injury when bending forward to pick up objects off the floor.

Tight hamstrings and parallel spine muscles restrict this pose, and may restrict seated sports, leading to lower back disc injuries. (Please note: If you have a disc injury, refrain from doing all stretches in this series except the Cobra.)

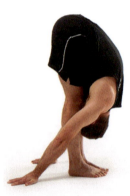

Forward Bend Standard

- Fold your trunk towards your knees
- Keep your legs straight

Stretch series for the Bear

Stretch series for the Bear

BEND STRETCH SERIES	REPS OR TIME
Forward bend	5 breaths
Hamstring stretch 3	1 min each side
Seated bend	1 min
Cobra	10 reps: exhale go up and go down when need to inhale

BEND STRETCH SERIES	REPS OR TIME
Child's pose	1 min
Downward dog	16 breaths

Movement and posture activation exercises for the Bear

We assign the ipsilateral crawl pattern and the bend pattern to the Bear. The ipsilateral crawl pattern invokes such survival reflexes as to move toward food or safety. It is linked to the adrenal glands and involves the same-side arm and leg moving together to propel motion. Babies perform a back extension as they prepare to stand—much like a bear raising itself onto its hind legs to shake a branch or warn off enemies.

Range of active movement exercises for the Bear

The Bear crawling pattern is an ipsilateral moving Downward Dog (*Adho Mukha Svanasana*), in which the legs and arms remain straight and the same-side arm and leg move at the same time.

Range of active movement exercises for the Bear

BEND MOBILITY	REPS OR TIME	TEMPO	ROUNDS
Bear crawls	x 10 forward and back	2 sec	1-3
"Y" Good mornings	x5 each side	2 sec down and 2 sec up	1-3
Situps	x 10 ea	1 sec forward and 1 sec back	1-3
Locust	Breathing pace	Inhale up and when need to exhale go down down 1-2 mins	1-3

Perform 1-3 rounds (one round is a completion of all 4 exercises).

Movement Stability and Yoga Balance

The Dancer balance pose (*Natarajasana*) is selected for the bend pattern because it activates the superficial back line and works in the opposite direction to the stretches.

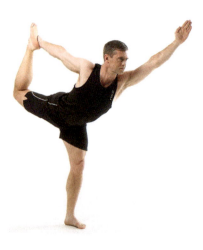

- Hold the balance for 5 breaths each side
- Repeat 1-3 times

After following this programme for four to six weeks, you will see a significant improvement in your range of bending movement and stability.

Why is the Bear the Power Animal of the bend?

The bear is a very strong animal that lifts itself onto its hind legs (as if performing a deadlift) to make a clawing gesture or shake trees. The deadlift and the snatch are active expressions of the posterior chain or superficial back line.

11. Push Like a Crane

The Crane   Front Arm Lines

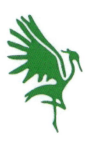
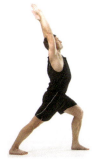
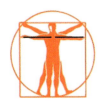

ROAM properties: Push

FASCIAL LINE	LIFE MOVE-MENT	FLEXI-BILITY	POSTURE	STABILITY	CRAWL	ANIMAL
Superficial and deep front arm	Push	Warrior I	Prone Cobra	Hand-stand	Single leg hip-hinge	Crane

Push activities include push-ups and bench presses, and daily motions such as opening a door or pushing a shopping trolley or a pram.

It is more common in sport and in daily life to perform single-arm pushes, such as throwing a ball or pushing a door, and therefore also requires help from the twisting muscles of the core and the opposite leg in a lunge pattern.

Pushing movement patterns use the chest and are usually coupled with lunge foot patterns. Restriction in the shoulder results from tight chest muscles and a tight thoracic spine, and this can lead to impingement injuries and restrictions in lifting objects above your head.

Fascial lines

The dominant fascial lines of the crane are the superficial and deep arm lines. The front functional lines used in pushing are assigned to the Crane.

Yoga flexibility pose assessment and standard

The Crane's asana and life movement is Warrior I and push. Warrior I (*Virabhadrasana I*) opens up the front line (back-leg top calf, back-leg hip flexor, abdominals, chest, and thoracic spine) and strengthens the front leg in a lunge pattern. The push muscles are the same muscles birds use to flap their wings.

The test procedure is simple: you either can or cannot do it to standard. If you cannot, this indicates that you require a period of restoration of range and stability of movement to regain function.

Warrior I tests the calves and the hip flexors of the back leg, the chest muscles involved in the ability to raise the arms and extend the upper (thoracic) spine backwards.

Most people—men, in particular—past the age of forty lack thoracic extension. Warrior I is not ideal for measuring this, as the body has many cheat mechanisms (whether conscious or subconscious) that hide areas of tightness. One giveaway is an excessive arch in the lumbar spine when lifting the arms above the head. If you are unsure, please double check this using the overhead squat test.

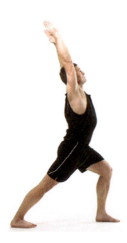

Warrior I Standard

- Keep back leg straight and foot facing forward
- Keep the font shin bone vertical
- Lift arms above the head
- Extend the torso (from the shoulder blades up) backwards

Stretch series for the Crane

PUSH STRETCH SERIES	REPS OR TIME
Warrior 1	5 breaths
Spine extension 2	2-15min
Upper traps	1 min
Calf Stretch	1 min each side

PUSH STRETCH SERIES	REPS OR TIME
Pec Major stretch	1 min each side
Hip Flexor Stretch	1 min each side
Standing hamstring stretch	1 min each side

Movement and posture activation exercises for the Crane

While this is not strictly a crawl, the Crane crawl pattern (*Urdhva Prasarita Eka Padasana*) is a single-leg hip-hinge moving-standing splits and single-leg hip-hinge type of exercise. It is not necessary to go to full splits—go to the active range of motion you can comfortably achieve. The Crane crawl resembles a crane sticking its beak into the water to catch fish. The single-leg movement can be used to help in push movements. Going into this crawl pattern is similar to swinging into a handstand and provides useful indication of when your wrists, elbows and shoulders are strong enough to support your weight.

Range of active movement exercises for the Crane

PUSH MOBILITY	REPS OR TIME	TEMPO	ROUNDS
 Crane hip walk	x 10 forward and back	2 sec down and 2 sec up	1-3
 Novice handstand	x5 each side	5 second hold Caution shoulder, elbow or wrist injury	1-3

ROAM: MOVEMENT AS MEDICINE **87**

PUSH MOBILITY	REPS OR TIME	TEMPO	ROUNDS
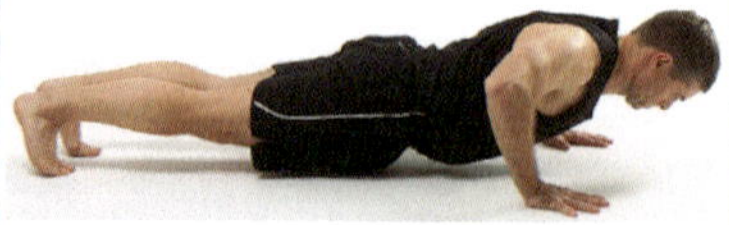 Push up side plank	x 10 ea	2 sec down and 2 second up and 1 sec pause in side plank (see picture below)	1-3
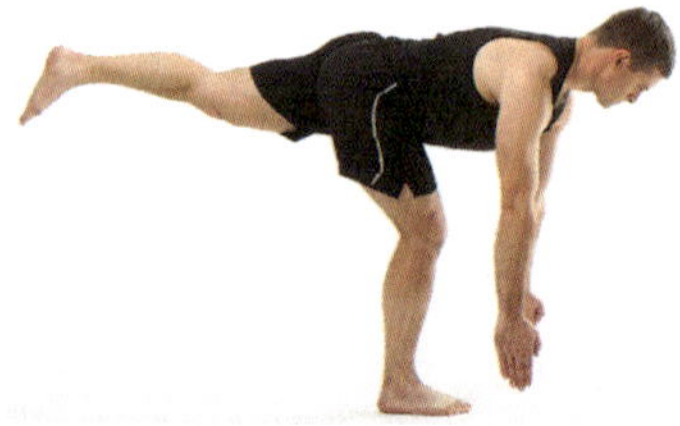 Single leg hip hinge	8-12 ea	2 sec down and 2 sec up	1-3
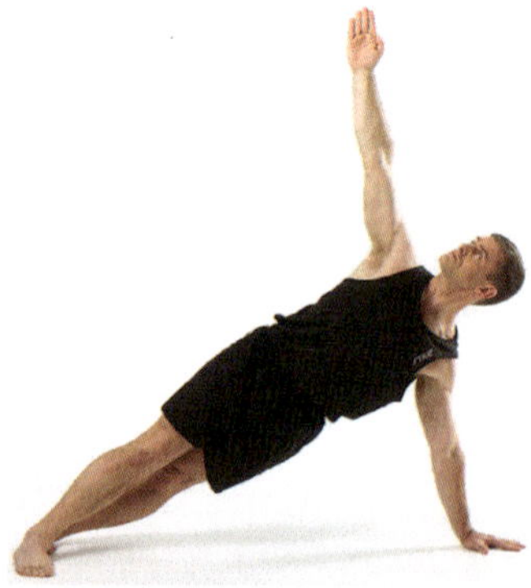 Side plank	Change when needed	Up to 70 seconds each side. Caution shoulder, elbow and wrist injury	1-3
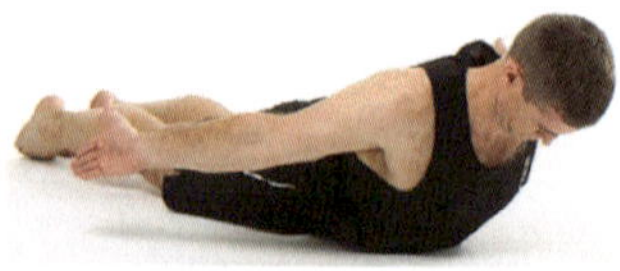 Prone cobra	breathing pace	Inhale up and when need to exhale go down 1-2 mins	1-3

Perform 1-3 rounds (one round being a completion of all 6 exercises).

Movement stability and yoga balance

The Crane's balance pose is the handstand (*Adho Mukha Vrksasana*). Mastering the handstand takes months, if not years, of practice. I have included it here because it engages the appropriate fascial lines, as well as to demonstrate that people require disciplined practice to achieve this goal.

If you have never previously done a handstand, if you have injured or weak wrists, elbows or shoulders, or if you have any other injury, please consult a professional yoga instructor or gymnastics coach to safely learn the handstand. Otherwise, stick to the novice handstand (as described above) until you can hold it for a full minute, or follow the progression described below..

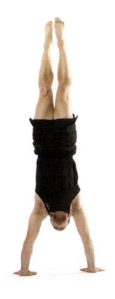

Basic progression:

a. Strengthen the wrists, elbows and shoulders through all the animal crawls and mobility exercises

b. Perform the handstand with your feet on a chair so you become used to inversion

c. Learn to safely twist or fall out of the handstand

d. Walk up the wall with your feet, with your stomach in

e. Once you've attained the handstand, build your tolerance to holding the position

f. Attempt to hold a freestanding handstand with a partner supporting you

My upcoming iPhone App *Bodyweight Ninja 90* includes a series of handstands and easier progressions to help you perform this difficult yet rewarding asana.

Why is the Crane the Power Animal of the push?

Although the Crane is not part of man's evolutionary chain, I have included it within the YogaVinQi Code to represent the pushing movement pattern, because flapping the wings requires very efficient and strong chest muscles. The push uses the chest and shoulder muscles. A crane will stand on one leg awaiting its prey and then dip its beak down to capture the prey.

The TCM meridian lines for the lung and large intestine have the same fascial arm lines as the push movement muscles. The associated Metal element's negative emotion is depression and its positive emotion is courage.

90 ROAM: MOVEMENT AS MEDICINE

12. Pull Like a Monkey

The Monkey Back Arm and lateral lines (as viewed from front)

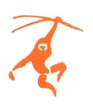
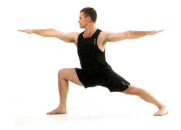
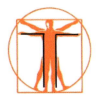

ROAM Properties: Pull

FASCIAL LINE	LIFE MOVE-MENT	FLEXI-BILITY	POSTURE	STABILITY	CRAWL	ANIMAL
Lateral Functional	Pull, Lunge	Warrior II	Alternate Superman	Tree	Lateral Hop	Monkey

We use the pull muscle to pull open doors, to perform pull-ups, and to bring anything closer to the body. Usually we pull with one arm and the opposite leg in a lunge pattern. This functional movement sequence involves the lunge in the pull (just as the lunge is involved in the push).

Fascial lines

The dominant fascial lines for the monkey are the back arm and lateral lines. The back functional line is also used in pulling and is assigned to the Monkey.

Yoga flexibility pose assessment and standard

The Monkey's asana and life movement is Warrior II (*Virabhadrasana II*) or the pull. Warrior II is a sideways pose that stretches the short and long groin muscles and strengthens the legs in a lunge pattern. The arms are held wide, as if you have just drawn a sword or are preparing to swing from one branch to another.

The test procedure is simple: you either can or cannot do it to standard. If you cannot, this indicates that you require a period of restoration of range and stability of movement to regain function.

Warrior II tests the muscles in the groin of the back leg and the hips of the front leg.

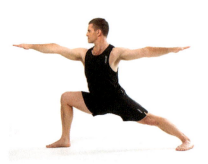

Warrior II Standard

- Keep the back leg straight with the foot turned out 45 degrees

- Front leg bent with shin bone vertical and thigh bone horizontal

- Trunk is vertical

- Arms are horizontal

Stretch series for the Monkey

PULL STRETCH SERIES	REPS OR TIME
Warrior II	5 breaths
Groin Stretch	1 min each
Straddle	1 min
Ql Stretch	1 min each side

PULL STRETCH SERIES	REPS OR TIME
Neck rotation	1 min each side
Gate	1 min each side

Movement and posture activation exercises for the Monkey

The Monkey's crawl pattern is the lateral hop, in which both hands and both feet hop to one side and acknowledges the sideways-oriented swinging movement and the ground-based movement patterns of apes. This hop pattern strengthens the wrists and shoulders in preparation for arm balancing.

Range of active movement exercises for the Monkey

PUSH MOBILITY	REPS OR TIME	TEMPO	ROUNDS
Monkey hops	5 forward and back	2 sec	1-3
Novice pullups	x 10 forward and back	2 sec down and 2 sec up	1-3
45 degree lunge	10 each side	10 each side	1-3

PUSH MOBILITY	REPS OR TIME	TEMPO	ROUNDS
 Bunny hops	5 forward and back	2 sec	1-3
 Alternate superman	1-2 mins	Inhale up, exhale down	1-3

Repeat 1-3 rounds. 1 round is completing all five exercises.

Movement Stability and Yoga Balance

Tree pose (*Vrksasana*) requires activation of the lateral line, as with any single-leg balance, and stretches the groin adductors that are stretched in Warrior II.

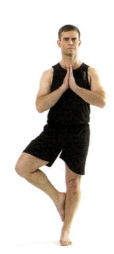

Tree pose is a one-legged standing pose, with the option for the hands to be positioned in prayer pose, at the heart or above the head. The legs represent the roots of a tree. The trunk of the body represents the trunk and the arms are the branches.

Why is the Monkey the Power Animal of the pull?

The term *brachiation* refers to the monkey-like movement of grabbing hold of something and pulling ourselves toward it (with one arm and the opposite leg forward; a lunge and pull action) as babies do when they are learning to stand. We use this movement on the gymnastics rings and the high bar, and when climbing a tree or a mountain, pulling open a door or paddling a canoe.

Vitruvian Man Linear Table

The table over page provides a summary of the five animals and the two "man" key movement qualities and abilities. Included is space to record your Power and Critical Animals for a ready reference to your exercise habit.

Vitruvian Man: Linear Table

SYSTEM	BEAR	MONKEY	DRAGON	CRANE	TIGER	MAN	PLAY
Fascial line	Backline	Functional Back	Lateral, Back arms, Back functional	Superficial front, Front arm	Deep front, Back functional	All	All
Movement	Bend	Pull, lunge	Twist	Push, lunge	Squat	Walk, run	Jump
Flexibility pose	Forward Bend	Warrior II	Revolved Triangle	Warrior I	Overhead Squat	Tadasana	Savasana
Balance pose	Dancer	Tree	Eagle	Handstand/ inversion	Warrior III	Tadasana	Savasana
Posture Pose	Locust	Alternate arm & leg raise	Horse Stance dynamic	Prone Cobra	Scarecrow	Stand wall lean	Standing Cobra
Crawl pattern	Straight arm and legs at the same time	Lateral hop	Wiggle	Single leg hip hinge	Contralateral	Inchworm	
Power Animal							
Critical Animal							

AUTHOR'S NOTE

Part I covers the systematic Western approach of how to identify and correct movement dysfunction by stretching tight muscles and activating weak muscles and then integrating this improvement into functional life movements.

The spiritual connection of roam and emotion.

The spiral symbol in the middle of the ROAM cycle represents growth in many indigenous societies as is present in many companies logos. For ROAM it represents the recommend way in which to develop your movement ability - that is grow from inside out in progressively increasing concentric circles. You will have noticed an emotion ring in the ROAM cycle; the emotion is the positive and negative emotion related to an element according to TCM. Originally there was a part II of ROAM, Movement as medicine but after consultation with various people I decided to cut it from this book to ensure the movement science was clear and concise. Part II is added to "Sort Your Life Out" is called "The YogaVinQi Code" and combines movement with the mind by adding in an intention to be mindful of when performing the exercises - the emotions are based on the 5 element theory. "The YogaVinQi Code" takes a step by step approach to unlocking the complex secrets of traditional Chinese medicine and yoga chakra theory to help heal physical-mental-emotional and spiritual trauma and point you in which of the four solutions may best help you feel better and start your health, fitness and performance journey from.

The four solutions.

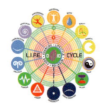

1. Life: "Love your Life"

"Sort Your Life Out" is the Lifestyle book that uses the Life Cycle as an assessment tool to direct you to one or more of the four solutions in more detail.

2. Intention: "Calm your mind"

"Calm Your Mind" is a book with many short and long term strategies to help you reduce depression or anxiety and get into the zone of optimal performance.

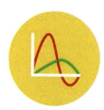

3. Food: "Eat Real Food"

"The Bottom Line of Fat loss" is a book that covers the ABC's of fat loss and critical information about nutrition and exercise.

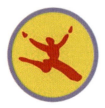

4. Exercise: "Enjoy Regular & Varied Exercise"

"ROAM: Movement As Medicine" provides the foundation of restoration movement and provides a platform for all the movement apps we have developed and "ROAM II: Function Meets Strength"; which adds multiple equipment modalities to ROAM to add huge variety to your exercise habit.

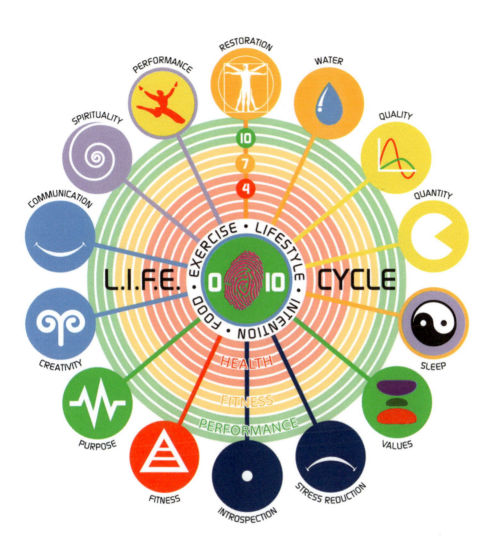

102 ROAM: MOVEMENT AS MEDICINE

BIBLIOGRAPHY

Byrne, Rhonda. *The Secret*. Atria Books 2006

Chang, Stephen T. *The Complete System of Self-Healing: Internal Exercises*. London: Tao, 1986.

Chek, Paul. *How to Eat, Move and Be Healthy!*. Chorley: C.H.E.K. Institute, 2004.

Eathorne, Ross. *How to calm your mind*. Self-published E-book on Kindle 2015.

Eathorne, Ross. *The bottom line of fat loss*. Self-published print book on Amazon and e-book on Kindle. 2016

Emoto, Masaru. *The Hidden Messages in Water*. New York City: Atria, 2005.

Gerber, Richard. *Vibrational Medicine: The #1 Handbook of Subtle-Energy Therapies*. Rochester: Bear and Company, 2001.

Hartley, Linda. W*isdom of the Body Moving: An Introduction to Body-Mind Centering*. Berkeley: North Atlantic, 1989.

Hawkins, David R. *Power Vs Force: The Hidden Determinants of Human Behavior*. London: Hay House, 2004.

Hébert, Georges. *Guide pratique d'éducation physique*. Paris: Librarie Vuibert, 1912. Translated by Pilou and Gregg. parkour.gr. Accessed May 4th, 2016. http://parkour.gr/books/physed-guide-hebert-nov09.pdf

Hoff, Benjamin. *The Tao of Pooh*. New York City: Penguin, 1983.

___. *The Te of Piglet*. New York City: Penguin, 1993.

Johnson, Jerry Alan. T*he Secret Teachings of Chinese Energetic Medicine, Volume 1: Energetic Anatomy and Physiology*. Monterey: International Institute of Medical Qigong, 2005.

___. *The Secret Teachings of Chinese Energetic Medicine, Volume 2: Energetic Alchemy, Dao Yin Therapy, Healing Qi Deviations, and Spirit Pathology.* Monterey: International Institute of Medical Qigong, 2005.

___. The Secret Teachings of Chinese Energetic Medicine, Volume 3: *Developing Intuitive and Perceptual Awareness, Energetic Foundations, Treatment Principles, and Clinical Applications.* Monterey: International Institute of Medical Qigong, 2005.

___. *The Secret Teachings of Chinese Energetic Medicine, Volume 4: Prescription Exercises, Healing Meditations, and the Treatment of Internal Organ Diseases.* Monterey: International Institute of Medical Qigong, 2005.

___. *The Secret Teachings of Chinese Energetic Medicine, Volume 5: An Energetic Approach to Oncology, Gynecology, Neurology, Geriatrics, Pediatrics, and Psychology.* Monterey: International Institute of Medical Qigong, 2005.

Kehoe, John. *Mind Power Into the 21st Century: Techniques to Harness the Astounding Powers of Thought.* Zoetic Books, 2007

Kendall, Florence Peterson. Provance, Patricia. McCreary , Elizabeth K. *Muscles, Testing and Function: Muscles testing and function: With Posture and Pain.* Lippincott Williams & Wilkins; 4th edition (January 1993)

Laughlin, Kit. *Stretching and Flexibility.* Simon & Schuester, Australia, 2000

Maclean, Paul D. *The Triune Brain in Evolution: Role in Paleocerebral Functions.* New York City: Springer, 1990.

https://en.wikipedia.org/wiki/Science_and_inventions_of_Leonardo_da_Vinci

Myers, Thomas W. *Anatomy Trains: Myofascial Meridians for Manual and Movement Therapists.* London: Elsevier, 2001.

Pottenger, Francis Marion. *Symptoms of Visceral Disease: A Study of the Vegetative Nervous System In Its Relationship to Clinical Medicine.* St Louis: CV Mosby, 1922.

"Science and inventions of Leonardo Da Vinci." Wikipedia. Accessed May 4th, 2016. https://en.wikipedia.org/wiki/Science_and_inventions_of_Leonardo_da_ Vinci

Simpson, Liz. *The Book of Chakra Healing.* New York City: Sterling, 1999.

Tzu, Lao, and Brian Browne Walker. *The Tao Te Ching of Lao Tzu: A New Translation.* New York City: St Martin's Press, 1995.

Made in the USA
Charleston, SC
17 June 2016